GET IT?
GOT IT.
GOOD!

Get It? Got It. Good! is every teenager's wellness encyclopedia.

Laura Martin, M.S. Ed. Health Educator
South Carolina Dept. of Health and Environmental Control

This type of publication is long overdue—by investing in our youth, ultimately, we will fulfill the goal of saving a generation.

Sharon Nelson, Director, New York City Partnership

Get It? Got It. Good! is the first book I have seen that really deals with the audience for whom it is targeted. It is an excellent supplement to curricular offerings and encourages teens to seek help from their families and community professionals.

Dr. Patricia Dignan, Superintendent

Get It? Got It. Good! is a book every teenager should read and share with parents. It serves as a valuable resource in my work.

Larry Warner, MA, LLP, Psychologist

Noël gives a realistic look at the rights and responsibilities and pleasures and pain of growing into adulthood. Not only do teens need to read **Get It? Got It. Good!**, but they'll want to.

Su Nottingham, Sex Educator, Teacher, Trainer

You can do anything if you put your mind to it. For me, that's the most important message in this book.

Jason, age 16

A GUIDE FOR TEENAGERS

GET IT?
WHAT YOU SHOULD KNOW

GOT IT.
WHERE TO FIND OUT

GOOD!
WHO TO TALK TO

Carol Noël

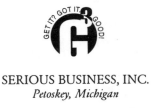

SERIOUS BUSINESS, INC.
Petoskey, Michigan

Published by Serious Business, Inc.
2909 Depew Road, Petoskey, Michigan 49770.

Publisher's Cataloging-in-Publication Data
Noël, Carol.
    Get it? Got it. Good!: a guide for teenagers / Carol Noël — Petoskey, Michigan. : Serious Business, Inc., c1996.
        p.   ill.   cm.
    Includes bibliographical references and index.
    ISBN 0-964947-0-0
    1. Teenagers—life skills guides. 2. Teenagers—Services for.   3.Teenag-ers—Services for—United States—Directories. 4. Teenagers—Conduct of life.
I. Title.
HV1431.N64 1996
361.8' 973—dc20   96-67556

PROJECT COORDINATION BY   JENKINS GROUP INC.

99 98 97   ❖   5 4 3 2 1

Printed in the United States of America

To Brad for his perpetual optimism, humor and love.
To Nick, Andy and Noel for giving as much patience
and encouragement as any working mother could
expect from her young children.
To Mom for her direct line to God.
I love you all.

United Nations Declaration of the Rights of the Child

- The right to affection, love and understanding.

- The right to special care, if disabled.

- The right to adequate nutrition and medical care.

- The right to protection against all forms of neglect, cruelty and exploitation.

- The right to learn to be a useful member of society and to develop individual abilities.

- The right to free education and to full opportunity for play and recreation.

- The right to be brought up in a spirit of peace.

- The right to a name and nationality.

- The right to enjoy these rights, regardless of race, color, sex, religion or social origin.

Contents

caine/crack. Heroin. Ecstasy. LSD. Speed. Steroids. The risks aren't worth it. Do you have a drug problem? Finding happiness elsewhere. Natural highs.

Preface

Don't look now, but you're in for the ride of your life. It's a time to discover who you are and what you want to be in this world. It's also a time to decide where you hang with drugs, sex and violence.

What's it going to be?

You can live your life with self-respect, forever friends, and a promising future. Or you can be miserable, failing in school, arguing with your parents, killing yourself with drugs and unprotected sex or spending time behind bars.

Life is precious. You can never get it back. So, don't lose it. Live it.

Arm yourself with knowledge. Knowledge is power. Make friends and be a friend. Determine your values and don't let anyone destroy them. Realize that decisions you make now may have far-reaching consequences. Know that if you stumble, it's just part of learning to walk in this world as an adult. Just as important, reach out to others when you need help. It's not a sign of weakness, but a sign of maturity.

Turn to your family first. They're the people who love you the most and will support you. If that's not possible, find someone else you feel comfortable with and who has experience helping kids your age: a teacher, counselor, priest, minister or rabbi, a relative or a trusted adult in your neighborhood. Get up the nerve to join a self-help support group in your school or community. Spilling your guts in front of other kids is hard, but dealing with your problems or worries face-to-face can be a powerful cure.

In this book, there are also names and phone numbers of reliable people and organizations which can lend as much support or as little as you want. They can also direct you to help in your own backyard. Be assured, your questions and needs will be kept private. These people don't care what your name is, where you come

from or whether you're rich or poor. They're only interested in helping you. They're not out to pass judgment.

The ride of your life should be rewarding and fun.
You can make it happen...but you have to learn the facts
before you act. If you're searching for answers to your
questions, turn to someone you trust, pick up the phone
or pick up this book.

I, too, had to search for answers and learn the "facts"
before writing this book. I succeeded by relying on my
own knowledge and experiences, pouring over countless
books and articles and turning to many talented and
generous people. People who willingly shared their ex-
pertise, their generousity, and their contagious devotion
to kids.

A sincere thank you to: Bob Goldberg, M.S.W.; Dr.
Robert Malachowski; Dr. Carl Taylor, Institute for Chil-
dren, Youth and Families, Michigan State University;
Jerry Berg and his Peer Counseling I,II,III groups; the
wise man in the Detroit airport; Kathleen Johnson; Bill
Geha, and his Toledo PRIDE support and leadership
groups; Su Nottingham; Vicki Vance; Irma Noel; Sharon
Nelson; computer wizard Debbie Adamski; Herman
Humes; Tulani Smith; Dr. Patricia Dignan; Mason
Buckingham; Community Strategies for Youth; District
Health Department #3; Dr. Gustav Lo; Probate Judge
Honorable Fred Mulhauser; Dr. James Scott Fleming;
DARE Officer Robert Voice; Paula Lacey; Judy Hardy; Toni
Felter and Charlie Bennett; Andrea Sterritt; Cindy
Okerlund; Carol Ann Harris; and Lori Chamberlain.

Applause, applause also goes to all of the kids in
Toledo, Petoskey, Charlevoix, Alpena, New York, Harbor
Springs, Los Angeles, Saginaw and Texas for sharing their
dreams and secrets with me.

At present, teenagers know little of the vast resources
available to them in their neighborhoods, cities, states
and country. Hopefully this book will bring together those
who have so much to give and those who are so wanting.
For, in today's world of easy-access information, there's
no excuse for ignorance. Get It? Got It. Good!

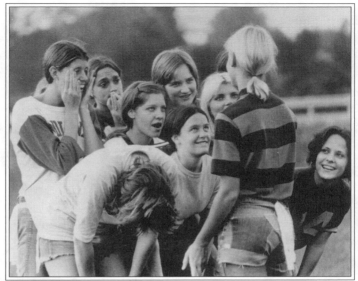

1

The World According to You

There is something I don't know
that I am supposed to know.
I don't know what it is I don't know,
and yet am supposed to know,
and I feel I look stupid
if I seem both not to know it
and not know what it is I don't know.
Therefore I pretend I know it.
This is nerve-racking

since I don't know what I must pretend to know.
Therefore I pretend to know everything.
I feel you know what I am supposed to know
but you can't tell me what it is
because you don't know that I don't know what it is.
You may know what I don't know, but not
that I don't know it,
and I can't tell you. So you will have to tell me
everything.

FROM KNOTS, R.D. LAING

Untying The Knots

I'm OK. I look good.
I have a good personality.
I'm not threatened by new people, ideas or situations.
I feel confident facing problems and making decisions.
I feel I have a lot to contribute to a relationship.
I'm worthwhile.

Do you feel this way about yourself? Or do you think these things are true only about other people you know? Do you suppose a person who feels this way has a pretty good life?

You can bet on it.

Anyone will tell you the best way to untie life's knots is through positive self-esteem. Life won't always go the way you plan and having confidence in yourself will see you through tough times. Feeling good and accepting who you are will also bring you more success in love and relationships, school, your job and whatever the future may bring.

Feeling Good About Yourself

I think having good self-esteem is very important.
As long as you like who you are, you can get
through anything.

JENELLE, 18

The great news is you, or anyone, can learn to have

positive self-esteem. The power to do so is within your-self and your way of thinking.

- First, be honest with yourself. Figure out what your strengths and weaknesses are. Try to get the most out of your strengths without demanding or expect-ing too much of yourself.

- Don't beat yourself up over your weaknesses, just work hard to improve yourself. Understand that self-esteem comes from living through both good times and bad. Facing bad times head-on can make you stronger, wiser and more self-assured. As Mary Pickford once said:

  If you have made mistakes, even serious ones, there is always another chance for you. What we call failure is not the falling down, but the staying down.

- Remember that one day may be far better than an-other. Take things one day at a time and just do your best.

- Give yourself a break. It's hard being caught be-tween childhood and adulthood. When you were young, other people made decisions for you. Now that you're older, it's up to you. This can be a drag sometimes, especially when you make a decision that is smart but not popular.

- Don't compare yourself to others or try to be what you think everyone wants you to be. Set goals and standards only for yourself and strive to reach them.

- Never say "never," "I won't" or "I can't." Saying things like, "I can't do anything right," or "I'll never be able to get along with my parents," often makes it come true. Be positive in what you think, say and do.

- Like yourself. You have to like you before others will.

Be In Charge

Life is 10% what happens to you and 90% how you react to it.

CHARLES SWINDOLL

Although self-esteem comes from within, we often let others shape it for us. Since you were born, you've been receiving a lot of messages, from a lot of different sources. Your parents, teachers, friends, TV, magazines and music have all been trying to tell you what to do and what not to do. Who to date. How to wear your hair and how to dress. Who to choose as friends.

Some of these messages are positive and helpful. They can teach you right from wrong. They can make you feel good about yourself and boost your sense of pride. But some of these messages can be negative and hurtful. So, anytime someone sends you a message, take charge of it.

- Look at the message clearly. What is it telling you to do? Buy a certain brand of athletic shoes? Be a perfect son or daughter? Get straight A's in school? Have sex before you're ready? Drink and drive?

- Does the message matter? Is the message reasonable? Does it fit with your own personal values? How does the message make you feel? Happy? Angry? Unworthy? Stupid?

- Confront the message and deal with it. Ask the person who sent the message how the situation could be made better.

- Make a change if you decide the message is helpful and is best for you.

- Don't get sucked in by commercials. Advertisers like to imply that a certain brand of athletic shoes will make you cool and powerful, but let's be real. They'll say anything to get you to buy their product and make them richer.

- Hang out with people who give you respect and understanding. Find a friend who asks, "Is something wrong? How can I help?" rather than, "You're wrong to feel that way."

- Remember, it's only a message. You have control over how it makes you feel. Don't let another person's unkind words or actions cut you down.

Someone might say:
"You shouldn't feel that way."

And your reaction can be:
"I shouldn't feel this way, but I do, so there must be something wrong with me."

Or:
"Until I can figure out a way to make the situation better, I am entitled to my own feelings."

If someone says:
"Come on, everybody's doing it."

Your reaction can be:
"If I don't do it too, people may not like me."

Or:
"I'm not everybody, and I know what's best for me. My true friends will like me even if I decide not to do this."

Your parents might say:
"Why didn't you get an "A" in that class?"

And your reaction can be:
"I have to be perfect all the time."

Or:
"I did the best I could this time. Next time I'll do things differently and try for a better grade."

Be your own best friend. Have faith in yourself...the way you look, act, think and feel. Nothing will help you through life more than believing you are a valuable person. As author John Naisbitt said:

Don't let the world inform you of whether or not you're happy, for heaven's sake, or whether you're of any personal worth. You get into big trouble that way, letting the world decide for you. You decide.

You Call The Shots

As a teenager, the responsibility to choose between right and wrong is now yours. Your parents are no longer constantly by your side, and your friends make many of their own decisions. And their decisions may or may not be good for you. Only you know what's best for you. If you let your friends steer you around, you'll never get where you want to go.

Life is going to offer you four choices: good, bad, hard and easy. It's easy to choose which movie to see, which sport to try out for, or which clothes to throw on in the morning. It's much tougher to choose between sex and abstinence, between soda and beer at a party, or between being like your friends or being your own person.

The best choice for you may be the hardest to make. It may help to remember that few things in life are free. It may be hard to wait to have sex, but think of the price you might pay: pregnancy, AIDS and heartache.

When the pressure is on to make a decision, have the courage to be an individual. You are your own person. You, and only you, will have to live with your decisions be they right or wrong. You must decide what to believe in and what you want to do.

Follow your own values. If you respect life, reject violence. If you admire honesty, always tell the truth. If you believe that knowledge is the key to a good job, stay in school. It's not always going to be easy to stick to your values, but you'll be happier for it.

If you find yourself struggling with some of life's decisions, look to your Mom or Dad, or a favorite teacher or counselor to help. Watch them. Question them. Learn from them.

Stress: Energy Or Enemy?

Are there days when you feel like being a teenager isn't all its cracked up to be? You're faced with sex and drugs and disease and school work and parents who expect a lot of you. It's enough to make anyone want to pull out all their hair, bite off all their nails, hide out for awhile, or sleep in all day.

You're stressed out. Everyone feels this way at one time or another. Stress is your body's way of dealing with pressure, threats and strain. It can keep you on your toes, motivate you and make you more alert. Or it can eat you up and spit you out. You can lose your energy, your attitude and your sense of humor. Stress may also be the bad guy if you have:

- headaches and tense muscles

- the feeling like a mac truck is sitting on your chest making it hard to breathe

- a loss of interest in school or work

- bouts of crying or anger you can't seem to control

- more arguments with your friends and family

- problems eating or sleeping (doing it too much or too little)

- a craving for alcohol or drugs

- a feeling of being rushed or pressured

- no energy

- an inability to relax and have fun

Get a Grip

You need to get a grip on your stress, instead of letting it get a grip on you.

- Keep in mind that most worries in life never happen, can't be changed, turn out better than expected or aren't really that important anyway.

- Make sure your worry is worth worrying about. You're not Superman or Wonder Woman, so ask yourself: "What can I control— my course load, my free time, how I feel about myself? What can't I control—my friend's mood, my curfew, the lousy weather? If you can control the situation, do something to change it. If you can't, move on.

- Figure out how really important the stressful situation is. Does it really matter that he or she doesn't like you? Will you go crazy without them? Is it really going to make a difference to the rest of your life? If the answer is "no," or "probably not," let it go.

- Close your eyes and imagine yourself in a favorite place having fun. Maybe you're hanging out at the mall, camping in the woods, shooting hoops, or going out on a date.

- List everything you're feeling stressed out about— your health, your family, your girl or boyfriend, your grades, your job, the future, war, the environment. Include even the smallest things that bother you. Then take one item at a time and deal with it. Come up with as many ways to handle your worries as you can.

- Learn how to deal with problems head-on. Holding in anger stresses no one but yourself. It helps if you set some goals, write a to-do list, then DO.

- Let your feelings out in a safe way. If the problem can't be solved right now, talk to someone you feel comfortable with. Go for a run. Hit your pillow. Write out your feelings. Remember, if the situation can't be changed, then change your attitude about the situation.

- Eat well, sleep enough and exercise. A healthy body makes a healthy mind.

- Ask a parent, school counselor, clergy person or teacher to help you get a grip.

- Lighten up! Get crazy! Have fun! Life's too short to be taken too seriously.

Highs And Lows

One day you feel up. The next day down. Welcome to the teenage years. A lot of things can go wrong in a day:

you're cut from a team, grounded, break up with your girlfriend or boyfriend, or fail a test.

Everybody hits the skids now and then. Depression is normal (eight out of ten teens say they've been depressed). It's not coping with it that spells trouble...

Are you:

- Not having fun anymore? Feeling like you could care less about school, friends, your future, your family?

- Withdrawing from friends or family; wanting to be alone? Feeling apart from your family? Not talking to your parents or arguing with them a lot?

- Feeling different than usual? Are you quiet rather than your usual open, friendly self?

- Eating or sleeping differently? Unable to sleep or sleeping a lot? Eating less or more?

- Having trouble handling a big change in your life: the death of a family member or friend, a divorce or break up of an important relationship, a move to a new city, a change of schools?

- Feeling sick or tired a lot?

- Using alcohol or drugs to make you feel better?

Depression can make you feel as if you have no control over the way things are, that life is hopeless. But you can help yourself.

- How are you looking at the world? You may think everything is going wrong, but usually a lot is going right, too. Don't give up. Focus on the positive.

- Ask for help from a friend, a parent, a school counselor, or a clergy person. Let someone help you find out what exactly is bothering you.

- Happier feelings often follow actions that make us happy. So, play ball. Check out a new movie. Buy a new CD. Cruise on the Internet. Hang with friends. Shop. Everyday do something fun and then increase the number of times you spend do-ing it. Try new things, too.

- Do your duties. If you have homework, do it—or you'll feel guilty. Count your victories, even the smallest ones, like getting out of bed in the morn-ing. Notice how often you win each day.

- Eat enough. Sleep enough. Get some fresh air.

- Get involved. There are so many worthwhile projects to choose from: Big Brother/Big Sister, the teen center, peer counseling, church activities, home-less shelters, soup kitchens, retirement homes, tutoring programs, special olympics, 4-H, scout-ing, MADD and SADD, to name a few. Check with your school counselor or the local Chamber of Com-merce. Helping others will make you feel stronger, happier and more confident. It's not only a great way to beat the blues, but to end boredom, too.

Depression: A Matter Of Life Or Death

I came close to committing suicide. I have the scars to prove it. They won't ever let me forget, but I don't want to. Since my attempt, I've had some of the best times of my life. I just wish it hadn't taken so much to convince me that life is worth living.

ELI, AGE 17

For Eli, suicide was not a problem, it was a solution. For a long time he had been depressed, feeling hopeless, helpless and alone. He tried to be happy, but "why bother." He "just wasn't worth it."

The only thing that saved his life was heroism—not on his part, but on the part of his best friend. What Eli attempted was not heroic. The reason he is alive today is because of the courage of his best friend who took Eli's threats seriously. Even though he had promised not to tell, he told Eli's mom about her son's plans. Together, they found him, near death, with only minutes to spare.

Some people become so overwhelmed with their prob-

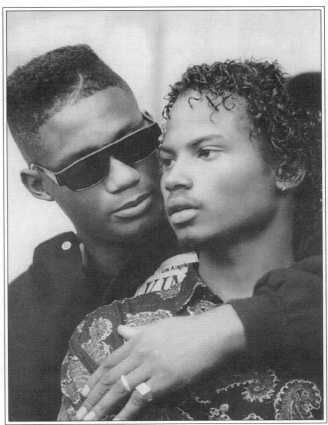

AP/Wide World Photos

lems, they decide the only way out is to take their own life. In fact, every six hours another American child dies at his own hands. Sadly, suicide is one of the leading causes of death for people between the ages of 15 and 19 years old.

Suicide never happens suddenly, although it often seems that way. The signs may be obvious or so hidden nobody realizes it until it's too late. Know how to tell when someone's life is hanging by a thread. People who need help often:

- have problems eating or sleeping
- withdraw from friends and family
- change the way they look or act in ways that might suggest an "I don't care anymore" attitude
- cry easily and often
- lose their temper more and pick fights
- make remarks like, "You won't have to worry about me anymore," or "My parents would be better off without me"
- get things in order and give valued objects away
- try to hurt themselves by abusing drugs or alcohol
- are unable to accept a recent loss
- become suddenly calm after a long period of depression as if they know the end to the pain is near
- do more than just think about it—they plan the suicide and the means to carry it out
- write poems, songs or letters about depression or death
- have attempted suicide before

People who are suicidal often have trouble sharing their feelings and believe no one understands them. They can and must be convinced through words and actions that they are worthwhile and help is available. And it is—for you or for someone you know through your parents, school, church or synagogue or community programs.

Reach out. There are lifelines all around.

Surviving A Loss

I hated him for leaving me. How could he be so selfish? If he was that stupid, he deserved to die. Oh my God, I don't really mean that. I loved him. I'll always love him. But I don't think I'll ever be able to understand.

SARAH, 16, A SURVIVOR

If someone who is thinking about suicide confides in you, here are some "do's and don't's" to help you re-open the door of life:

DO	DON'T
Take all threats seriously.	Don't take a threat lightly.
Always be interested and sincere.	Don't try to analyze the person.
Be firm. If you think the person needs counseling, tell them, don't ask them.	Don't promise confidentiality. It's okay to violate a friend's confidence when it's done to save a life.
Ask questions. "Have things ever been this bad for you?" and "Are you thinking of hurting yourself?"	Don't argue the pros and cons of suicide (there are no good reasons for it).
Stay with the person if there is immediate danger.	
Always be willing to seek professional help.	

There are hundreds of thousands of attempted suicides every year. Every completed suicide leaves survivors feeling angry, sad and guilty. They're mad at the person who committed suicide, at the fact that it happened at all, at the doctor who couldn't perform a miracle, at parents, friends, at the whole world, and even at themselves. If only they had listened more... loved more... known more... Remember, if the survivor had been in control the other person would still be alive.

In the case of a suicide, get to know the facts. Rumors can fly after a completed suicide. Don't defend or glorify the reasons behind the act. There is no problem so big it's worth the taking of one's own life.

Grieving

If you have survived a loss due to death, divorce or the breakup of an important relationship, grief is a natural and healthy reaction.

Everybody's different, but the process of grieving can last a long time. It may take one to several years to cope with everything that's going on in your heart and mind.

Your first reaction is going to be one of denial and shock: "This can't be true! Everything was fine yesterday." Then you might feel sad, angry and ashamed all at the same time. You'll cry for your loss. You'll want to scream at the person who left you. In death, you may feel ashamed you're still alive and even believe you are somehow responsible for what happened. It's not unusual, either, if you find yourself making promises to be "good" in hopes that it will bring the person back.

It's important to release your feelings. Let go. Talk and talk and talk some more—with someone who cares— a neighbor, friend, family member or counselor. And if it feels right, cry long and hard. It's not babyish. It's a very natural way of relieving pain.

Before it's all over, you'll fight exhaustion and depression. You may not be able to concentrate on your studies, a close relationship, sports or other interests.

Be patient with yourself. Time is a great healer. Your grief will come to an end, and both your love for that person and your life will carry on.

Remember the "whole" person, as he or she was in life, not in death. Keep a journal. Record important dates, and do something special in that person's memory.

No matter what the loss—a parent, friend, sibling or pet—you are the same person you were before. You can let the loss strangle you or make a promise to yourself to be happy. You may not be able to change what happened, but you do have the choice and the power to overcome it.

The best thing you can do is take care of yourself. Keep busy, eat well, exercise. Go to church. Get professional help. Help others through their grief; it will lift your spirits, too.

Divorce: After The Breakup

Nobody died, but divorce can make you feel as if they did. The two people in this world who taught you how to love now say they don't love each other. They promised to be together forever—now your parents are splitting up.

"What in the heck are they doing?" you ask, and "Where does this leave me?"

Though you'd probably like to send them to their room until they work the whole thing out, that's probably not an option. So, the next most important step is to realize it's not your fault. Don't blame yourself. And don't lay the blame on only one of your parents: "It takes two to tango."

- Remember that while you're tangled up in your own feelings about your parent's breakup, they, too, are grieving over the loss of their marriage. They may not be able to rise above their own heartache to show they still care for you. At times, you may feel as if you've been left out in an orbit on your own.

- It's okay to cry and be angry, but don't let these feelings control you. Don't divorce your parents after they divorce each other. Don't lash out and make matters worse by fighting, coming home late or failing classes. It will only make your life more miserable.

- Don't play the middleman and don't take sides. Don't carry messages, rumors or angry words back and forth between your mom and dad. Sometimes it may seem as if your parents are fighting about you. More than likely though, they're really fighting feelings of disappointment, anger, sadness and guilt over their failed marriage. They may even still love each other and have trouble letting go.

- Stay involved with both parents, if possible. Work at being close even though you are separated. Be the first one to reach out your hand if you must. Try to share your feelings with your parents, knowing full well that you both have needs. Openly showing your love and concern will help the whole family survive the loss of the relationship. Most importantly, it will assure your parents that they haven't lost you as well.

- Talk to another adult you trust. You'll feel better if you can share your thoughts and feelings.

- Understand that life is going to change, and there probably isn't anything you can do to stop it. Don't try to get your parents back together like in the movies. You'll be in for a big let down.

- If you have the painful decision of deciding who to live with, choose what's right for you. Your parents are old enough to take care of themselves.

- Take care of yourself and your own needs during this family crisis.

Losing a parent through divorce need not mean the death of the family. You are still the same person. Your parents are still the same people you know and love. Divorce may shake the relationship you have with them, but it doesn't have to destroy it.

Cinderella And Snow White

Cinderella and Snow White haven't done much to help the stepfamily business. Not being able to party at the ball or being served poison apples is a drag, but neither happen very often in real stepfamilies.

A stepfamily is different and takes some getting used to. There's no such thing as love at first sight. You may have to move to a new home, make room for new brothers and sisters or meet new grandparents. You may have to switch back and forth between your mom's house and your dad's. A stepparent may change house rules or take part in disciplining you.

Expect a little frustration and confusion. Things are going to be upside down for awhile. You may have to change plans, ideas and schedules, so that everyone's needs are met. But a lot can be gained if you give it a chance, so hang in there.

Be fair. Your new stepparent may not be your birth mom or dad, but may have special qualities of their very own.

Keep an open mind. You may hate the fact that your new stepbrother wanders into your room without permission. But, who knows, maybe a little unexpected company isn't so bad after all. If you want to put the brakes on him, do it nicely. It's the best way to get someone to do what you want and to respect your wishes.

You may always love your real mom and dad more than a stepparent. That's normal. If you do form a good relationship with your stepfamily, great! Don't feel guilty. You're not being disloyal. You have a heart big enough to love a lot of people.

Stay in touch with grandparents, cousins, and favorite aunts and uncles on both sides. Keep the lines of communication open to help heal the family and keep everyone together.

Talk with someone who is not related to you if you feel you need some unbiased advice.

On The Run And Homeless

If you run away, try to get help; otherwise, what's the point. You should do something to make it better.
BEN, 16

You just can't take it anymore. Life is too tough at home. So, you run and think your story will have a happy ending. Not likely.

Take it from teenagers who know (there are one million who try running every year): "It can be a big bad world out there."

There are a lot of reasons people run away from home: personal problems, difficulty at school, abuse, or a bad relationship with parents or family members. The real reason, though, is the person feels they can't solve their problems any other way.

Unfortunately people who run from their problems find even bigger ones on the run. It's hard to make friends. It's hard to know who to trust. It's tough to find a job or a safe place to live. Most of all, making a home on the street can be dangerous. The longer you're gone, the greater the chance you'll be the target of a violent crime, sex and drug abuse, pregnancy and disease.

Most runaways find out early that it's far better to work out problems while living at home. In fact, most of them return home within three days of leaving.

If you're tempted to run or know someone who is, try to talk your problems out with your parents and family or a trusted adult. Teachers, counselors and youth workers at runaway shelters may also be able to help you find a better solution.

Some kids find themselves out on the street because of a family breakup, abuse, the loss of a job or a lack of money. This doesn't have to mean they're without hope. If you need counsel, food, shelter or clothing, check with the youth center, local health department or runaway shelter in your town.

Before you have to test your muscle alone on the streets, use your strength and smarts to find help and solutions at home.

Making The Best Out Of Bad Situations

Life can be tough. No one can promise it will always be fair. Bad things do happen, but they don't last forever.

Each time you're faced with a challenge, learn from it. The more experience you have solving problems, the easier it gets. Here are some of the best ways to go from bad to better.

- Hang in there. If you're in a bad situation, get through it as best you can. When it's over, look back, learn and come up with better ways to handle the same kind of situations in the future.

- Don't start asking yourself, "Why does this always happen to me?" This kind of attitude is self-defeating. Be realistic. First, it probably doesn't always happen to you. Secondly, whatever the problem, there are always other people who have been there, done that, and come out okay. You're not alone.

- Exit. Sometimes the best thing to do is walk away from a situation. Deal with it when you've cooled off and can look at it with a more level head.

- Redirect. Find something else to take your mind off the problem or disappointment.

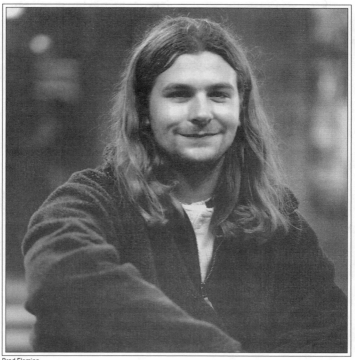

Brad Fleming

- Divide and conquer. Sometimes we can get over-whelmed by a problem. Divide it into small pieces and deal with each a little at a time.

- Take a mental stroll. If you can imagine yourself working out the problem to your satisfaction, it can help spark new ideas.

- Deal with it. As often as possible, face the problem directly. Get it settled, so it won't bother you any longer.

- Get help. Two heads are better than one. Turn to someone who is responsible like your parents or teachers.

- Give yourself a break and don't be too hard on yourself. Take it one step at a time.

Remember, life is what you make it.

Reach Out

When your self-esteem needs a boost, there are a lot of people out there who can and want to help—your best friend, a favorite teacher, the school counselor, your mom or dad, your friend's parents or a clergy person.

If the blues keep hold of you for longer than a month, it's a good idea to talk to a professional. Open up—let them know how you're feeling. Let them help you help yourself. If growing up is what you're in the process of doing, remember, reaching out and talking to someone is, in fact, one of the most adult things you can do.

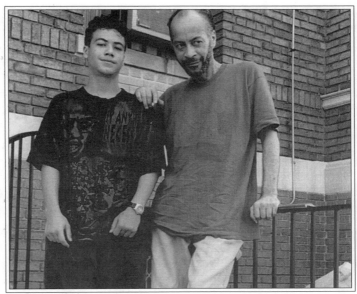

Nancy Shia, Impact Visuals

2

On The Level

News flash: Children were heard from around the world today when the Alien Research Division of the U.S. Defense Department announced that parents are human.

"No way!" cried one 15-year-old. "I can prove my parents are weird."

A spokesman for the defense department was also quoted as saying, "Contrary to what everyone believes, parents may not know every little thing about raising children and sometimes make mistakes. They also can't read their kids' minds, even though they've been trying to for years. This means that future generations of parents and teenagers will have to start talking with each other to keep their relationship from being lost in space."

Unfortunately, that's easier said than done. When any two people communicate, there is:

- What you wanted to say.
- What you meant to say.
- What you said.
- What you think you said.
- What the other person heard you say.
- What the other person thinks he or she heard you say.
- What the other person thinks you meant to say.
- What the other person feels about what you said.
- What the other person says about what you said.
- What you think the other person said about what you said.

Is it any wonder misunderstandings happen?
AUTHOR UNKNOWN

There's a lot to be gained from talking with your parents. When you talk—really talk—with them, you're showing them love and respect, and giving them a chance to show you love and respect in return.

Here's a little test that might help get the conversation going. (No fair asking your parents for the answers.)

What is Your P.I.Q. (Parent I.Q.)?

1. If your parents won the lottery, what would they do with the money: put it in the bank, travel or buy a new house?
2. Where was your mother born? Your father?

3. What kind of relationship did or do your parents have with their parents?
4. What kind of grades did your parents get in school?
5. What sports did your parents play while growing up?
6. Who is your mother's best friend? Your father's?
7. Do your parents believe in God?
8. What do your parents love most about you?
9. What do your parents like to do in their free time?
10. If your mom or dad could have any job in the world, what would it be?

Now, check your answers with your parents. If you got them all right, you're one smart kid. If you missed four or more, ask your parents for help. (And, from now on, take time to do more than yell, "Hi Mom," Bye Mom," "Hi Dad," "Bye Dad," as you go in and out the front door.)

Good Relationships Don't Just Happen

I get along great with my parents. In fact, my mom is my best friend. I know some of my friends think that's pretty strange, but, well, I think I'm lucky.

CAROL, AGE 15

Getting to know your parents, and vice versa, will help improve your relationship with them. But good relationships don't just happen. They take time, effort, patience and a lot of "leveling" on both sides.

How To "Level" With Your Parents

To "level," you have to be open, trustworthy, respectful and, sometimes, even quiet. Here's how:

- Talk about your feelings. Tell why you feel the way you do. They can't read your mind and won't understand unless you tell them. For example, "It hurts when you criticize me because I feel like I can't do anything right."

Not Helpful: Blaming other people for what is happening. For example, "You're always on my back for something. It's your fault we have all of these problems."

- Make sure what you say and how you feel are understood. Parents don't always "get it" the first time you say it. For example, "Mom, I'm not saying I can't ever do anything right. I'm saying that's how I feel when you criticize me."

Not Helpful: Jumping to conclusions and attacking. For example, "That's all you ever say. You're driving me crazy."

- Make sure you understand what is being said. Repeat what you hear to make sure you get it right. For example, "Are you saying you don't want me to stay out late because you're worried something bad will happen to me?"

Not Helpful: Being defensive. For example, "But everybody stays out late. Why do you want to be so mean to me?"

- Ask questions when you're not sure what's being said. Parents don't always get it out right, either. For example, "Dad, I'm not sure I understand what you're saying."

Not Helpful: Storming off angry. For example, "Well, just forget it. I know you don't trust me."

- Try to understand and check out how your parents feel. For example, "Mom, I hear you saying you are really afraid I will get pregnant."

Not Helpful: Name calling. For example, "Well, you're just being stupid. You're crazy."

- Ask your parents to listen. Set aside a time when you are most likely to have their full attention. For example, "Mom, there is something I want to talk about. Do you have time to listen?"

Not Helpful: Interrupting, talking too long. For example, "I don't care about that. You've got to let me do this because blah, blah, blah...."

- Respect their values so you can help teach them to respect yours. For example, "I understand getting an education is important to you, and you don't want me to skip school."

Not Helpful: Being critical of their beliefs. For example, "Oh, that's ridiculous. No one believes that."

- Look for other ways to agree. There are some things on which you and your parents can compromise on or meet halfway. For example, "Dad, I understand you're just not willing to let me do that. Could we talk about finding another way that might work for both of us?"

Not Helpful: Being sarcastic, condescending, or smart-alecky. For example, "Oh, that's silly. That would never happen to me. Yeah, right, I'm going to go out and smoke dope tonight, sure."

- Put yourself in their shoes before you act. What would you say to your kid? Maybe you'll decide not to act, or at least be better able to accept the consequence of your actions.

- Give reasons why. If you can explain why you do what you do, it might help your parents understand a little better.

- Control your nonverbal behavior, your tone of voice and facial expressions. Don't give mixed messages. When your words are loving but your voice is angry, what should your parents believe?

- Say you're sorry—and mean it.

- Share hurt feelings before they get too big to handle.

- Listen—don't interrupt. You hate it when they do it to you, so don't do it to them.

- Be honest.

- Show your parents you care about what they say and feel.

- Ask them what they think.

- Be open to their side of the issues.
- Avoid doing things which will stop the conversation. Keep your cool. Don't threaten, beg, argue, talk back or stomp off.
- Don't expect total agreement, but go for understanding and respect.

Leveling isn't easy—but the results are worth the challenge. If you have a relationship of mutual respect with your parents, you have it made. If you don't, give it a try. The relationship you build with your parents will have a lifelong effect on the relationships you have with your friends, your husband or wife and even your own children.

A Word To Parents—A Stage Of Predictable Confusion

Anna Freud, daughter of Sigmund Freud, and a pioneer in child psychoanalysis, aptly captured the reality of the teenage years when she said, "It is normal for an adolescent to behave for a considerable length of time in an inconsistent and unpredictable manner."

Parents of teenagers would say that's an understatement. Teenagers would say they're just "misunderstood."

What parents and teens both need to remember is given a mentally healthy and well-functioning environment, most adolescents are hopeful, positive and enjoy a loving relationship with their family.

In a healthy family system, there is mutual respect between parents and their kids. Parents allow some freedom to their teenagers and acknowledge them when they make a good decision. The more the child behaves responsibly, the more freedom they get. When teenagers are dealt with this way, parents are often pleasantly surprised. They may end up with a young adult who is different from what they pictured—but better—because the teenager had some hand in shaping his own identity.

The manner in which an adolescent goes about shaping his own identity often translates into predictable confusion for the entire family. The rapid changes in clothes, music and hairstyles is a way for the adolescent to say, "I am me. I am autonomous. And I'm going to make it really obvious I'm not you."

"At any given time," said Anna Freud, "a normal teen will love his parents and hate them; revolt against them and be dependent upon them; be deeply ashamed to acknowledge his mother before others, and unexpectedly, desire heart-to-heart talks with her; thrive on imitation while searching for his or her own identity; and be more idealistic, artistic, generous and unselfish than he will ever be again, but also the opposite—self-centered, egocentric, and calculating."

Now is not the time to force the adolescent into a predetermined mold. Building a healthy adult is a lengthy process and should start when the child is young. The younger the better. Trying to make a teenager be what you want him to be is like trying to force toothpaste back into the tube.

If you have a young teenager at home who is entering the "unpredictable" phase, don't be surprised or label it as abnormal. Despite their occasional unpredictability, teenagers aren't any different than the rest of us. We all are highly motivated by a little TLC (Tender Loving Care). And teenagers will identify with you, want to please you and incorporate your values as their own, with just the right amount of loving attention.

Loving attention can come in many forms—but one of the most important is communication—what you say to your son or daughter, how you say it, or saying nothing and just listening (when you're dying to scream).

Given enough patience and practice, knowing what to say, how to say it and when to listen can be learned. But first you'll need to take the time to really know your child and what he or she responds to positively.

Some Advice From Your Kids

According to some teenagers, showing you love them is just as important as saying it. Their advice to parents:

"Kiss me on the cheek."

"Take me out to lunch with you."

"Joke with me."

"Watch football on TV with me."

"Sit down and talk with me."

"Teach me how to cook."

"Don't let me get away with everything."

"Be open-minded."

"Be supportive."

"Trust and respect me."

"Listen to me."

"Take time to really get to know me."

What Is Your C.I.Q. (Child I.Q.)?

Rush, rush, rush. Clock in. Clock out. Drive your kids around. Fix dinner. Clean up. Check homework. Fall into bed. Parenting leaves little time for really knowing your child. This test will help you discover just how much or how little you know about your son or daughter.

1. Who is your child's best friend, and why?
2. What would your child do with $10?
3. Does your child believe in God?
4. What is your child's favorite subject in school? Favorite teacher?
5. What does your child like most about you?
6. If your child could do anything on a Saturday afternoon, what would it be: go to the mall, play sports or watch TV?
7. What does your child want to be when he or she grows up?
8. What is your child's favorite food?
9. Who does your child admire or idolize?
10. What would be your child's ideal birthday? Who would they invite? What would they do? What gift would they like the most?

Check your answers with your child. If you scored a perfect "10," you have earned the "Parent of the Year" award. If you missed four or more. take some of the rush out of your day to spend more time getting to know your child, and then take the test again.

Educate Yourself—Then Educate Your Children

I'm lucky because I have a caring and supportive family. My parents feel they have a responsibility to know what is going on in my life. Although I may resent it at times, I know they are just worried about me and want what's best for me.

SARAH, 16

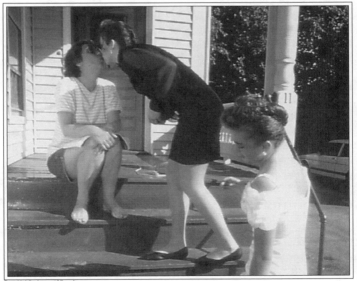

Dan Habib, Impact Visuals

Once you realize your child is more than a bunch of hormones with skin pulled over it, try to discover more every day. Talk to your child about day-to-day events. Lay the foundation, so they'll find it easy to come to you with problems.

Besides learning more about your own child, educate yourself on drugs, alcohol, sexual issues and teenage depression. Don't assume that because your son or daughter doesn't ask you questions about these sensitive subjects, they aren't curious or don't have problems. Your silence conveys the message that they're not supposed to ask you questions, so they often find the answers elsewhere. (And there are a lot of unreliable sources around.)

You may be scared to start talking about some of these issues with your kids. What parent isn't? What if just talking about sex or drugs encourages them to try it?

Rest assured. Research conducted by the World Health Organization and the Centers for Disease Control and Prevention shows, for example, that sex education works to delay or decrease teenage sexual activity and makes them more responsible. It also is most successful when given to kids before they begin sexual activity.

If you want to, bring up the subject yourself. Be creative. Use items from the news or themes from TV shows to bring up the subject. Be an "askable" parent. Keep the lines of communication open. Respond to questions when asked. Be clear and honest and tell it like it is. Don't use scare tactics or fables. Most importantly, be comfortable with these issues yourself, so you can approach them with a level head.

Communicating Love

There are many ways you can show loving attention toward your child and encourage two-way communication and respect.

- Talk with them as you would like them to talk with you. Be consistent in the way you communicate with them.

- Listen. If your mouth is open, your ears aren't. Put down the newspaper, ignore the phone, stop what you're doing. Look at your child directly in the eyes and really listen for as long as it takes.

- Ask again if you don't understand the first time.
- Explore together mutual alternatives on issues for which compromise is acceptable.
- Don't be afraid to admit you don't know or you made a mistake.
- Stay calm. Yelling raises everyone's defenses.
- Avoid using expressions like "Where did we go wrong?" "When I was your age . . ." "After all we've done for you . . ." or "You'll get over it." All these do is make your child feel guilty and insignificant.
- Don't underestimate or minimize the intensity of your children's feelings.
- Give reasons for your behavior to help them better understand why and how you acted in a certain way.
- Control your nonverbal behavior, your tone of voice, your facial expression —don't give potentially mixed messages. Your child will always pick up on the negative one. A furrowed brow or crossed arms implies that you've already made up your mind before hearing the whole story.
- Watch for the message behind the words. Look for nonverbal cues that might tell you more about how your child is feeling.
- Say you're sorry—and mean it.
- Avoid doing things which will bring conversation to a halt. Everybody loses if you threaten, plead, lecture, probe, argue, overanalyze, belittle, talk back, interrupt or walk away.
- Don't let hurt feelings fester. The longer harm stews, the more damage it does.
- Be in touch with your own feelings and know your

children have a right to their own and they may be different from yours. You don't have to agree all the time. A good relationship is also possible when everyone involved can sometimes agree to disagree.

- Give your emotional support.
- Maintain confidentiality—teach trusting ways.
- Be honest.
- Show your children you care what they say and feel. Put yourself in their shoes. Ask them what they think and be open to their side of the issues. If you want your child to act respectably, you must show them respect.
- Help your children set realistic goals.
- Praise your children. Catch them doing something right!
- Show confidence in them.
- Don't expect total agreement; rather, go for understanding and respect.
- Keep your sense of humor. Laughing with your child is a great way to break down barriers.
- Stand by your child when they are upset or are working out a problem. Avoid taking on their feelings, pitying them or pushing them into a solution prematurely. LISTEN . . . REFLECT . . . LISTEN, believe in their abilities to solve their own problems with your support and guidance.
- Don't try to convince your kids you're perfect. It's too great a shock to them when they find out you're not.
- If problems arise that are too hard to handle, don't be afraid to seek advice and counsel from someone both you and your child respect and can relate to.
- Show your children you care by teaching them local emergency numbers. Use the space provided in

the back of this book to write the numbers down for future use, and provide medical authorization in case emergency care is needed.

Children Learn From Watching You

Ideal parents not only raise their kids but also act as role models, friends and supporters. The best parents discipline in a positive manner. They try to understand their child's mistakes and help her to grow and become a stronger person.

TIFFANY, 17

Every time you communicate with your children and show them your affection and attention, you are, in essence, telling them what you value in life and giving them guidelines for creating their own values. You shape their lives with every word, every touch. You are their role model. Children learn to love, lead, problem solve and achieve from you.

Remember, too, it's sometimes more important to let them find their own way. Your children need to experience cold, fatigue, adventure, injury, risk, challenge, failure and frustration to learn, feel, change, grow, love and live.

It takes a lot of time and courage to pursue—and keep pursuing—a good relationship with your child. Let them know you love growing with them. Let them know you look forward to knowing them as adults—when they'll not only be your child, but your friend.

Start talking now. The longer you wait, the bigger the gap between you, and the faster life passes by.

20 Memos From Your Child

1. Don't spoil me. I know quite well that I ought not to have all I ask for. I'm only testing you.

2. Don't be afraid to be firm with me. I prefer it; it makes me feel secure.

3. Don't let me form bad habits; I have to rely on you to detect them in the early stages.

4. Don't make me feel smarter than I am; it only makes me behave stupidly big.

5. Don't correct me in front of others if you can help it; I'll take much more notice if you talk quietly with me in private.

6. Don't make me feel that my mistakes are sins; it upsets my sense of values.

7. Don't protect me from consequences; I need to learn the painful sometimes.

8. Don't be too upset when I say "I hate you"; it isn't you I hate but your power to thwart me.

9. Don't take too much notice of my small ailments; sometimes they get me the attention I need.

10. Don't nag; if you do, I shall have to protect myself by appearing deaf.

11. Don't make any rash statements; remember that I feel badly hurt and let down when promises are broken.

12. Don't forget that I cannot always explain myself as well as I should; that is why I am not always accurate.

13. Don't tax my honesty too much; I am easily frightened into telling lies.

14. Don't be inconsistent; that completely confuses me and makes me lose faith in you.

15. Don't tell me my fears are silly; they are terribly real and you can do much to reassure me if you try to understand.

16. Don't ever suggest that you are perfect or infallible; it gives me too great a shock when I discover you are neither.

17. Don't ever think it is beneath your dignity to apologize to me; an honest apology makes me feel so surprisingly warm toward you.

18. Don't forget how quickly I am growing up; it must be very difficult for you to keep pace with me, but PLEASE TRY!

19. Don't forget I love experimenting; I couldn't go on without it, so please put up with me.

20. Don't forget that I cannot thrive without lots of understanding and love but I don't have to tell you that, do I?

AUTHOR UNKNOWN

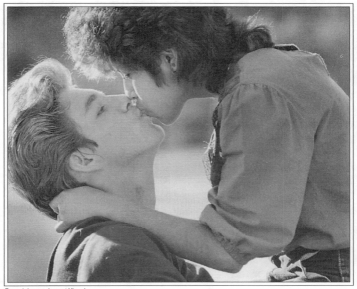
Evan Johnson, Impact Visuals

3

Facts And Fantasies

There are always going to be changes happening in your life, although it seems between the ages of 10 and 16 it's more intense. All of a sudden, you feel different, act different, think different, look different.

Powerful things called hormones may send you on a physical and emotional roller coaster. You grow hair, breasts or experience erections. You wear makeup, start dating and "get" your older brother's and sister's jokes. You notice how a classmate's hips sway when he or she walks down the hall. Your friends, hair styles and clothes change.

47

You Fall In Love For The First Time

It's not the same as loving your parents or your friends. Being in love can make you feel wild and crazy. It can also rattle your brain, making you believe that love conquers all. Well, love can do some pretty amazing things, but it won't cure pregnancy or AIDS. Did you know:

- Each year, 30,000 girls under the age of 15 become pregnant.

- Every year more than 1,000,000 girls between the ages of 15-19 become pregnant, and nearly half of them give birth.

- By age 18, one in four teenagers will become pregnant at least once.

- Fifty percent of sexually active teenagers say they don't use condoms or other contraceptives (birth control methods) the first time. Twenty-five percent of sexually active teens say they never use any.

- Almost 20 out of 100 teenage pregnancies occur within one month of first intercourse.

- Teenagers have the highest rate of sexually transmitted diseases than any other age group. Twelve million new sexually transmitted infections occur every year, 9 million of those affect men and women under the age of 25.

- A teenager contracts a sexually transmitted disease every 13 seconds (even from people they love).

(SOURCE: ALAN GUTTMACHER INSTITUTE)

These Aren't Fear Tactics, They're Facts

So, before you do it, wonder about it, or worry about it, get the facts. Educate your mind. Base your decision to have sex on reality, your own instincts and your honest answers to these questions:

- Do I really want to have sex? Why? Is it love or just a "crush"? Am I rebelling against my parents?

Do I just want to be able to "fit in" and tell my friends I have done it? Am I afraid my partner will break up with me if I don't? Do I think it will make me more of a man? More of a woman?

- How does the decision to have sex fit with my moral beliefs and values?

- How will I feel if my parents find out?

- Who is going to make sure we have the best birth control and are using it the right way?

- What am I going to do if a pregnancy happens?

- Do I want to wait until I'm married?

- How many people has my partner had sex with? Is there a chance he or she might be carrying a sexually transmitted disease (STD)? How can I be sure they will tell me the truth about their past? Can I trust my partner? Can I trust my partner's other partners? What happens if I catch an STD? Could I die?

It's great to fall in love and want to express it. It's another thing to want to express that love in a risky way. If you think you're mature enough to have sex, then you also need to be mature enough to talk about important issues that will affect you both. If you're not ready to talk, you're not ready for sex.

So, before you do anything, talk openly with your partner. It's probably going to be tough. You may feel embarrassed. But the consequences of doing without talking can be much worse...

- If you think having sex means you'll be "together forever," but your partner still feels free to be a "player"—you'll feel hurt, angry and jealous.

- If your partner is immature or uncaring about sex— you'll hear and FEEL the rumors in the way other people treat you.

- If you think sex is going to make you more of a "real" man or more of a "real" woman, you may be surprised.   What it might really make you is a young, unprepared parent or a very sick kid.

- If your partner has a sexually transmitted disease (STD), like HIV/AIDS, herpes or gonorrhea—there's a good chance you'll catch it. (Guess what? You're not invincible.)

- If you don't use birth control or use it the right way—you or your partner may get pregnant and then be faced with sharing the legal and financial responsibilities of raising and supporting a child.

- If you're a teenage parent, you're more likely to be a high school drop out and less likely to complete college.

- Most teenage parents don't have enough money to support their new family and find themselves living in poverty.

- If either of you feel weird or guilty about having sex —instead of bringing you closer together, it can actually drive you apart.

Fact Or Fantasy?

Take this test by answering true or false to the following statements, and find out how much you really know about sex.

You can't get pregnant the first time.	T	F
You can't get pregnant standing up.	T	F
Condoms are 100 percent effective against pregnancy and disease.	T	F
You can't get pregnant if you withdraw before having an orgasm.	T	F
Taking one birth control pill before sex will prevent pregnancy.	T	F
Parents don't understand or care about sex these days.	T	F

Taking a hot bath right after sex will prevent pregnancy.	T	F
You can't get pregnant during your period.	T	F
Sharing a pack of pills with a friend will protect you both from pregnancy.	T	F
If you love another person, you can only prove it by having sex.	T	F
The pill prevents sexually transmitted diseases (STDs).	T	F

If you answered true to any of these statements, you need a crash course on the facts of life. Keep reading and take a lot of notes. If you marked every answer "false," congratulations for knowing the difference between fact and fantasy.

Follow Your Instincts

If you're thinking about having sex—but you have some doubts—no matter how small—WAIT. Any doubts you feel beforehand may leave you feeling angry, guilty and resentful afterwards. If you feel deep down you're not ready—listen to that voice. You have the rest of your life to be sexually active; don't let anyone rush or pressure you.

The best contraceptive devices are your feelings, your values, your beliefs, the facts and your instincts. Base your decision on these things, not on: your sexual urges, ignorance or pressure from friends. (The truth is—even though it may sound like a lot of your friends are having sex, almost half of those who say they are really aren't.)

And don't wait until the going gets hot to start talking. Your body can be your own worst enemy. Once turned on, it may be hard to break away from your sexual urges. But remember, you control these urges—not the other way around—and the final decision to have sex is yours and yours ALONE.

Your future doesn't just happen to you. You MAKE it happen with every big and little decision you make.

It's your body.
It's your life.
It's your decision.
Make the right one.

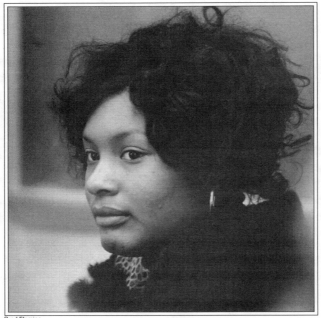
Brad Fleming

Don't Let The Pressure Get To You

"If you won't have sex with me, you don't really love me."

"If you won't have sex with me, I'll find someone who will."

"It will bring us closer together."

"Everybody's doing it."

"Nothing bad will happen."

"But I want to show you how much I love you."

"We'll be together forever."

"I promise you won't get pregnant."

"I promise I'm clean."

Professions of love? No way. These are the oldest lines in the book. They're threats and bribes and lies. Don't fall for them. The person who says them has only one goal: to pressure you into sex.

"He was touching me, and I couldn't move. I was afraid to stop him or act like I didn't want to. But I hated it. Why was I letting him do this? When had I decided that he was more important than I was?"
MELISSA, 15

If you decide not to have sex with someone, it should be enough to just say, "I don't want to," or "I don't feel comfortable doing that," or "I'm not ready." If being honest about your feelings is NOT enough, that should be a strong hint for you to take more time making your decision or find a new love interest.

Pressured sex isn't loving sex. It's possible to love someone without having intercourse. If your partner lashes out at you when you refuse to have sex, they are simply reacting to the blow to their ego.

If you really like the person, tell him or her you're not rejecting them, you're just not ready. Be assertive, and be a broken record. Even if you have to repeat these lines over and over again, your partner will eventually get the message.

"I feel just as strongly about you as you do about me, but if I can wait, you can wait."

"I don't have to prove my worth or my popularity by having sex. I have plenty of confidence in myself."

"If you love me, you'll respect my desire to wait."

"If I wanted to do it, I wouldn't be fighting about it with you."

Use
THIS REVOLUTIONARY 100% GUARANTEED METHOD
to
PROTECT YOURSELF
from
AIDS, CHLAMYDIA, SYPHILIS, GONORRHEA, HERPES,
and more.

VIRGINITY

To
USE IT, YOU DON'T HAVE TO PAY FOR CONFIDENTIAL TESTING,
embarrassing
APPOINTMENTS OR PILLS. IT'S FREE. AND YOU CAN DO IT
yourself
IN THE PRIVACY OF YOUR OWN HEART AND MIND
where
ALL THE DECISIONS THAT CAN CHANGE YOUR LIFE FOREVER ARE
made.

Virginity.
It's
worth it.

"I can live without someone who tries to force me into something I don't feel is right."

"I'm worth the wait."

"I'm not ready for marriage or a baby, and I don't want to risk it."

"I don't always agree with what my friends do. Anyway, it's their business, and this is mine, and I've decided to wait."

"I said 'NO,' I meant 'NO,' and that's the end of the conversation."

The decision to have sex has nothing to do with age. It has everything to do with your values and maturity. It's an understanding that you are responsible for your actions and your actions have consequences. It is also an awareness that a good relationship is about love and friendship, not just sex. It's a respect for the facts, your partner and yourself.

When it comes to sex, you need to think with your head—not your heart—especially in this day and age when more kids are having babies, catching STDs and dying from AIDS. You have the right to answer honestly, the right to refuse and the right to stand up for yourself.

When "No" Isn't Enough

He was so nice. I felt really comfortable with him. But one minute he was just standing there talking to me, and the next minute he tackled me, pinned me on the bed, and then he....

KIM, AGE 18

Sex without consent is a crime. Any act which forces someone into sexual contact through violence, threat or dishonesty is considered rape—even if you know the person—even if it's someone in your family, a relative or a friend of the family. In fact, rape by someone you know is more common than rape by a stranger.

Rape can be tried in a court of law. If you have sex

with someone after he or she has said "no," you may be found guilty as charged. In many states, sex crimes are legally tried as "criminal sexual conduct" (CSC), and the maximum penalty ranges from two years to life in prison.

So, Listen Up . . .

- Have you ever heard the old saying, "Their lips were saying 'no', but their eyes were saying 'yes'?" Well, listen up—no matter how shyly or quietly your partner says it, "No" means "NO."

- Talk to each other and set limits before you get into the heat of the moment. Decide together how far you are willing to go.

- If your partner is considered underage by state law (and state laws vary), you can be tried and convicted on criminal sexual conduct charges. Jilted friends and angry parents can prosecute you, even if your partner consented.

- Don't put yourself in a position where you'll be forced to "put on the brakes." If you keep finding yourself in these situations, find someone else who respects your feelings and values.

. . . Speak Up . . .

- Tell the person how all of the pressure is making you feel. He or she can't read your mind.

- If he or she continues to come on to you, get mad. Turn your fear into anger. Your own aggressiveness can help back down your aggressor.

- Determine how you want to be treated and stand up for that whether you are a male or a female. You are an important, worthwhile person with feelings and rights.

- If your partner can't hear you, be assertive. Look

the person in the eyes, say exactly what you mean and keep saying it over and over again.

- Don't giggle while saying "No" and let the person continue to come on to you. Say it like you mean it, and back up your words with body language.

- Pay attention to what your instincts are telling you. Even when someone grabs, tweaks or touches your privates, it can make you feel violated. If your date sits too close, blocks your way and seems to enjoy your discomfort, be on the alert. If the situation seems dangerous, GET OUT—even if it means being embarrassed.

- Try to decide the safest way out. Some girls fight, scream, tell the person they have AIDS, throw up, act retarded or pretend to faint. There's no one perfect way to prevent rape, and there are never any guarantees.

. . . And Don't Set Yourself Up

People who have this kind of forced sex on their mind are going to look for ways to get you alone, where you won't attract attention or be interrupted. By following these rules, you can reduce your risk of date rape.

- Know your date as best you can. If it's a new relationship, avoid being totally alone until you know he or she can be trusted.

- Be careful about using alcohol and other drugs. They can make you do things you normally wouldn't do and make you less able to resist. Keep an eye on your partner's use, too. Alcohol and drug abuse affects judgment in all of us.

- You may think being drunk gives you an excuse for not being responsible—but you made the decision to take the alcohol or drugs—so YOU are still responsible for what happens. Stay in control.

- Remember, rape is an act of aggression, not passion or love. The person doesn't love you—and he or she won't afterwards. If they loved you, they wouldn't force you.

- Most date rapes involve alcohol. In a court of law, a jury won't show much support for people who have placed themselves at risk by drinking or drugging.

- If a person continues to do things you don't feel good about, get rid of them. Cut that person from your circle of friends.

If You Are Raped

Get help right away! It is not your fault. Speak up.

- Go to a safe place.

- Do not shower, bathe or douche (spray water or other solution into the vagina to clean the area). Do not wash your hands, brush your teeth, use the toilet, change or destroy your clothing, or clean up the area where you were raped. You may be destroying evidence.

- Call the police and report the crime.

- Get medical attention as soon as possible. Go to a hospital emergency room for care. The hospital will use a "Rape Kit" to collect evidence in case you want to file criminal charges. The police can be notified from there.

- Talk to someone you trust right away, whether it be your parents, a teacher, counselor, friend or call a 24-hour rape crisis line. Coping with your feelings after being raped is as important as making sure you're okay physically.

- Be checked to make sure you're all right—that you're not pregnant or infected with an STD.

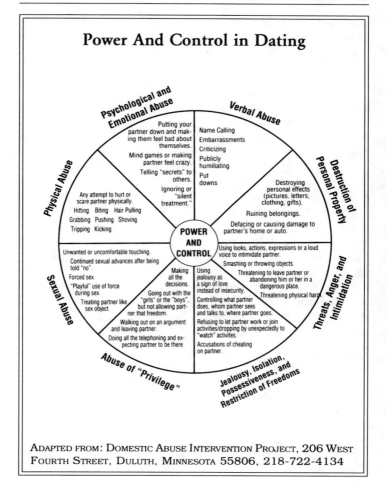

Power And Control in Dating

Psychological and Emotional Abuse
Putting your partner down and making them feel bad about themselves.
Mind games or making partner feel crazy.
Telling "secrets" to others.
Ignoring or "silent treatment."

Verbal Abuse
Name Calling
Embarrassments
Criticizing
Publicly humiliating
Put downs

Physical Abuse
Any attempt to hurt or scare partner physically.
Hitting   Biting   Hair Pulling
Grabbing   Pushing   Shoving
Tripping   Kicking

Destruction of Personal Property
Destroying personal effects (pictures, letters, clothing, gifts).
Ruining belongings.
Defacing or causing damage to partner's home or auto.

POWER AND CONTROL

Sexual Abuse
Unwanted or uncomfortable touching.
Continued sexual advances after being told "no".
Forced sex.
"Playful" use of force during sex.
Treating partner like sex object.

Abuse of "Privilege"
Making all the decisions.
Going out with the "girls" or the "boys," but not allowing partner that freedom.
Walking out on an argument and leaving partner.
Doing all the telephoning and expecting partner to be there.

Threats, Anger, and Intimidation
Using looks, actions, expressions or a loud voice to intimidate partner.
Smashing or throwing objects.
Threatening to leave partner or abandoning him or her in a dangerous place.
Threatening physical harm.

Jealousy, Isolation, Possessiveness, and Restriction of Freedoms
Using jealousy as a sign of love instead of insecurity.
Controlling what partner does, whom partner sees and talks to, where partner goes.
Refusing to let partner work or join activities/dropping by unexpectedly to "watch" activites.
Accusations of cheating on partner.

ADAPTED FROM: DOMESTIC ABUSE INTERVENTION PROJECT, 206 WEST FOURTH STREET, DULUTH, MINNESOTA 55806, 218-722-4134

Being Abused Without Being Touched

Physical abuse is only one way someone might force you to do something you don't want to—like having sex. If someone you love puts you down, calls you names or

constantly criticizes you, it's abuse. If that person threatens you, isolates you from family or friends, or tries to
control your every move, it's abuse.

Anyone can be an abuser—people you love, even
people in your own family: parents, brothers or sisters,
stepparents, relatives, live-ins and friends of the family.

No matter who the person is, don't let anyone abuse
you physically, sexually or emotionally. It doesn't matter
how much you love them, they have lost control of their
feelings and behavior and are using you as a target.

No matter what happens, no one has the right to treat
another human being that way, and you shouldn't give
them that right. Your life is worth more. Take a stand!
Speak up! It's not your fault. No one deserves abuse.

Find someone who can give you the strength to get
out of a bad relationship. Your school counselor, family
doctor and the people at the local health department or
Department of Social Services are always willing to help.

Remember, though, being abused is not something
to joke about. You should never lie about abuse or use it
to hurt someone. False accusations can ruin another
person's entire life.

Protecting Yourself

*My family went out of town at spring break, and
when I got back home, my girlfriend and I were
really excited to see each other. I had a condom, but
we started up before I had the chance to put it on. I
told her I would pull out before anything happened,
and I figured, what could happen just this one short
time? Now she's pregnant, and I'm not even out of
high school . . .*

DAVID, AGE 17

Choosing not to have sex is the only sure way of not
becoming pregnant or contracting a sexually transmitted disease. If the decision to have sex has already been
made, you CAN and MUST protect yourself to avoid these
lifelong consequences. It's not hard to do.

Ways to Express Love And Affection Without Having Sex:

Say thank you. Be honest. Share feelings, hugs and kisses. Watch a sunrise or sunset together. Make a surprise picnic. Listen carefully to positive and negative feelings. Give two or more compliments per day. Hold hands. Invite and pay for breakfast or lunch. Make a small or big photo album. Use magazine pictures to make a funny book about a shared experience. Give balloons. Put secret notes in secret places. Go to church or youth group together. Don't verbally attack the person. Do a drawing or make a card. Take a walk together and share the moment. Phone just to say you care or "I love you". Bake a cake or something the person likes. Go on a boat ride. Plan a surprise birthday party. Plan a "you're great" party. Buy or make a personalized t-shirt. Take a class together. Learn about something the other person really enjoys. Invite the person to a movie, play or concert. Make an ice cream sundae. Buy a little something you know that person would like. Invite the person to go to a dance. Volunteer to do something with that person's friends. Learn information about sex and sexuality from parents or someone you can trust. Share sexual feelings and values—and say "NO" if that's how you feel.

Adapted from material by Helena B. Valenzuela, MI Dept. of Social Services, Newaygo Intermediate School District.

Learn as much as you can before you do anything. The more you know, the less at risk you are.

Talk with someone. Your parents, for one. (They had you didn't they? They must know a little something about sex.) Though you may be scared to talk with them, you might be pleasantly surprised at their reaction. There are also experienced doctors, school counselors and youth workers who can and want to help you make the right choices. (Think before relying on your friends for the facts. Half of them may not be doing what they say they are and may not know as much as they say they do.)

One of the things you should know is that it isn't enough to just use birth control. You have to use it the right way. Did you know:

- Condoms may start to break down if kept in a wallet too long or in the glove compartment of a car on a hot summer day.

- Natural sheath condoms can help prevent pregnancy but may not protect you from all sexually transmitted diseases, including AIDS.

- Oil-based products such as Vaseline®, used as a lubricant, can break down the materials which make up diaphragms and condoms.

- Condoms are made by humans and used by humans, so they don't always work.

Another bit of advice you should know is: never rely on anybody else—including your partner—to use the right protection. Thinking that protection is only *her* responsibility or only *his* is wrong. It takes two. At the very least, it takes you. YOU PROTECT YOU.

The purpose of the following information on birth control and sexually transmitted diseases is to educate you, NOT to give you permission to have sex. At the very best, it will convince you to wait before jumping into behavior which is both dangerous and complicated.

What Is The Best Way?

The best way to protect yourself depends on:
- how often you have sex
- what you're comfortable using
- what is most safe and effective
- what you can afford

Every contraceptive method is different in both effectiveness and cost. The most important thing is to use a method which protects both of you from unwanted pregnancy *and* disease—and to use it every time.

The following list outlines various methods of contraception: how they work, how well they work and what they can mean to you.

Method: Abstinence

Effectiveness: 100%; works all the time, every time. No one has ever gotten pregnant or caught an STD from abstaining (not having sex).

How it works: partners agree to not have sexual intercourse.

What you should know: no cost and no side effects; no risk of getting STDs, Pelvic Inflammatory Disease or pregnant; meets the values of religions and churches when used before marriage.

Possible problems: none, but it may take willpower.

Method: Cervical Cap

Effectiveness: 73-92%; 10-25 women out of 100 will get pregnant in a year's time.

How it works: rubber, thimble-shaped cap, filled with spermicide, held in place over female's cervix by suction; fitted by a health care provider; cannot be worn during menstrual cycle; must remain in place 6-8 hours after intercourse.

What you should know: can be worn for up to 24 hours.

Possible problems: may be hard to fit; may cause urinary tract infections; may develop allergy to rubber or spermicide; damage to cervix or vagina may occur from cup rim pressure or wearing too long; possible risk of toxic shock syndrome (this disease, which is an infection usually linked to the misuse of tampons, can cause high fever, skin rash, nausea and vomiting, and sometimes death).

Method: Condom (rubber)

Effectiveness: 88%; out of 100 women using a condom during each act of intercourse for one year, 10-15 will become pregnant (this number decreases to 5 to 10 when spermicidal foam is used with a condom).

How it works: a close-fitting piece of thin rubber that fits over (is unrolled onto) the erect penis leaving 1/2" at the tip; may be used with a water-based lubricant; should be used with spermicide and other contraceptive methods; must be used only once.

What you should know: latex condoms (not natural sheath) lower the risk of spread of STDs as well as pregnancy (look for the word "latex" on the package); low cost; can be purchased without prescription; works best when used with spermicide (nonoxynol-9 kills sperm).

Possible problems: may affect sensation in males; may develop allergy to rubber; condom may break if damaged; may not protect against all STDs.

Method: Depo-Provera

Effectiveness: 99.7%; less than 1 woman out of 100 will get pregnant in a given year with Depo-provera.

How it works: a birth control method (given as a shot) which prevents the release of an egg from the ovaries during the menstrual cycle—if an egg is not released, it cannot be fertilized by sperm and result in pregnancy; one shot in buttock or arm prevents pregnancy for 3 months; requires reinjection every 12 weeks (more than 2 weeks late for follow-up shot may result in pregnancy); to avoid giving the shot during pregnancy, the first one must be given during menstrual period, unless the female is currently on birth control pills; must be given by health care provider.

What you should know: protects against pregnancy for 12 weeks; may take 12-18 months after last shot to become pregnant; reversible; convenient; cannot be removed from body; private.

Possible problems: side effects, which may decrease over time, include irregular menstrual bleeding, an increase or decrease in bleeding or no menstrual period at all, weight gain, headache, nervousness, stomach cramps, dizziness, weakness or fatigue, decreased sex drive and increased risk of developing osteoporosis (thinner bones); does not protect against STDs; initial costs may be high if PAP (pelvic) and breast exams are needed.

Method: Diaphragm

Effectiveness: 82-98%; as many as 19 women out of 100 will become pregnant in a given year (usually because the diaphragm is not used correctly every time).

How it works: rubber disc with flexible rim 2-4" in diameter, used with spermicide and inserted into the vagina, stops sperm from fertilizing the egg; fitted by a health care provider; must remain in place 6-8 hours after intercourse.

Possible problems: can be uncomfortable if not properly fitted; may cause bladder infection; may develop allergy to spermicide or rubber; doesn't protect against STDs.

Method: Female Condom

Effectiveness: 74%; approximately 25 women out of 100 will get pregnant in a given year using this form of birth control.

How it works: used by a woman in her vagina to block semen; must be used only once.

What you should know: can be put in place well before intercourse.

Possible problems: may not be as effective as the male condom for protecting against STDs; costs more than male condom; may develop allergy to rubber.

Method: Fertility Awareness Method (F.A.M.)—Rhythm; Basal Body Temperature; Mucous Method

Effectiveness: 75-97%; 10-25 women out of 100 will become pregnant in any given year.

How it works: different ways of checking the female body to determine fertility (the peak time for pregnancy to occur each month). The idea is to avoid intercourse during the fertile days; instructions must be given by a professional or successful, experienced user; depending on method, temperature and cervical discharge (mucous) must be checked every day and records kept to determine time when fertile.

What you should know: no side effects; no cost after method is learned.

Possible problems: must have agreement and support of partner; not always reliable—stress or illness and some medicines may change temperature and mucous; higher risk of pregnancy; doesn't protect against STDs.

Method: IUD

Effectiveness: 95%; 5 women out of 100 will get pregnant using an IUD for a year.

How it works: small, flexible, plastic device inserted by a health care provider into uterus for an extended period of time.

Possible problems: may increase menstrual cramps and blood flow; may cause pelvic infection; increased health risk if pregnancy occurs (possibility of tubal pregnancy in which the fertilized egg begins to grow while in the fallopian tube instead of the uterus); body may reject and expel IUD; doesn't protect against STDs; expensive.

Method: Norplant

Effectiveness: 99+%; less than 1 woman out of 100 will become pregnant in a year.

How it works: six small, thin flexible capsules filled with a hormone called progestin are inserted under the skin in the female's upper arm; minor office procedure to insert and remove capsules; requires yearly exam with pap smear.

What you should know: capsules provide constant birth control 24 hours after insertion; provides contraception for as long as 5 years; reversible.

Possible problems: side effects can include irregular menstrual bleeding, headache, nausea, nervousness, dizziness and weight gain; doesn't protect against STDs; removal is reported to be painful; insertion and removal are reported to be expensive.

Method: Pill (oral contraceptive)

Effectiveness: 98%; out of 100 women using the pill as directed for one year, 2-4 will become pregnant.

How it works: a synthetic hormone in the form of a pill is used by female to stop ovulation; must have a prescription to buy; regular checkups and PAP tests with health care provider are required.

What you should know: easy to use; may regulate periods and reduce menstrual cramps and flow; may lower the risk of ovarian cancer.

Possible problems: possible increased risk of heart attacks, strokes, blood clots, gallbladder disease and liver tumors (these risks are higher for smokers on the pill); does not prevent the spread of STDs; minor side effects may include slight bleeding between periods and nausea; must take pill every day; costs involve an initial physical exam and monthly payments for pills.

Method: Spermicide

Effectiveness: 79-97%; 10-25 women out of 100 will become pregnant in a given year.

How it works: foams, creams, jellies or suppositories with a chemical that kills sperm; placed into vagina with finger or applicator 10 to 30 minutes before each act of intercourse; should be used with other form of contraception.

What you should know: lubricates the area; may protect against STDs and Pelvic Inflammatory Disease; low cost, easy to use and no prescription is needed.

Possible problems: may develop allergy to spermicide.

Method: Sterilization

Effectiveness: nearly 100%.

How it works: surgical removal of part of the reproductive system; available for both male and female.

Possible problems: does not prevent STDs; reversal is possible but rare; costs more for females than males.

Method: Withdrawal

Effectiveness: 20-25%; approximately 75 women out of 100 will get pregnant in a year's time.

How it works: male withdraws penis from vagina and genital area before ejaculation.

What you should know: no cost.

Possible problems: male may release sperm before orgasm; opposed by some religions; doesn't protect against STDs.

Certain birth control methods are available without a prescription at the drug store. Other methods, such as birth control pills, require a yearly pelvic examination and pap smear in order to get a prescription for them.

If you don't know what to expect, pelvic exams may be uncomfortable (not painful), but they can be easier if you relax. The exam involves a health professional using an instrument called a speculum. A speculum looks a little like a duck's bill and helps to open the vagina to get a closer look inside. At the same time, a pap smear can be done to test for STDs, cancer or other problems in the vagina and cervix.

Male or female, if you are having sex, it's good to have regular checkups by a doctor or other health care provider every year. If your behavior places you at high risk for disease or pregnancy, you may even want to be checked more than once a year.

Many problems can be controlled or cured if found and treated early. And before you start worrying about whether you can afford all this, shop around. There are a lot of health clinics and agencies who offer checkups like this, and they really vary in cost.

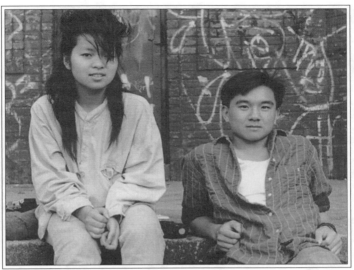

Arvind Garg, Impact Visuals

STDs: The Dangers Of "Doing It"

Test your STD and AIDS I.Q.

You can get an STD from deep, wet kissing.	T	F
You can have STDs or AIDS without knowing it.	T	F
The letters AIDS stand for Acquired Immune Deficiency Syndrome. HIV stands for Human Immunodeficiency Virus.	T	F
Taking illegal drugs can increase your chance of getting an STD.	T	F
STDs can be passed back and forth between partners.	T	F
Latex condoms with the spermicide nonoxynol-9 should always be used for safer sex.	T	F
Condoms have a 15% failure rate.	T	F
Once you have HIV, you have it for life.	T	F

You can have HIV for up to 10 years or more without getting AIDS.	T	F
Since 1985, all blood transfusions have been screened for HIV.	T	F
Having HIV is not the same as having AIDS.	T	F
Having one STD puts a person at higher risk for getting others.	T	F
AIDS and STDs can be prevented.	T	F
AIDS and STDs can happen to anyone, even you.	T	F

The answer to every one of these questions is "true." How well did you do? If you got some wrong, read on and take the test again after finishing this chapter.

What Are STDs?

Sexually transmitted diseases are infections of your sexual and reproductive organs. They can be spread through close sexual contact such as intercourse, oral and anal sex, and/or the exchange of body fluids like blood, semen and discharge from the vagina.

STD germs live in warm, moist areas like the mouth, rectum and genitals. Some STDs, like herpes, can even be contracted by kissing someone who is infected. Yet, kissing is still one of the safest ways to physically show your affection for someone.

Sometimes painful, and even deadly, STDs are often silent. A person can be infected without knowing it and then turn around and infect their partner.

The Symptoms Of STDs

Any one of the following symptoms could be a clue something is wrong:

- Discharge from the penis or vagina that's not normal in consistency (texture and feel), smell or color
- Deep abdominal or stomach pain

- Pain or bleeding with intercourse
- Sores, bumps or blisters near the genitals or mouth
- Burning or itching around the female's genitals
- Flu-like symptoms with fever, chills and aches
- Pain when urinating
- Rashes on the body
- Swollen glands

The following list tells about different kinds of sexually transmitted diseases: their symptoms, how they are spread, treatments and what can happen if they're not treated or cured.

STD: Chlamydia

When Symptoms Appear: 1-3 weeks or longer after being infected.

Symptoms: often none; in men—watery to creamy discharge from penis, burning and swelling in testicles and itching around opening of penis; in women—burning with urination, bleeding/pain with intercourse, lower abdominal pain, bleeding between menstrual periods.

How Contracted: vaginal, oral or anal intercourse.

Cure: blood test is needed for diagnosis; partner must also be tested and treated; antibiotics are used for treatment; shouldn't have sex until completely cured.

What Can Happen If Not Treated Or Cured: sterility (an inability to have children), PID (pelvic inflammatory disease), pneumonia or eye infections in newborns following vaginal delivery.

STD: Gonorrhea (Clap/Drip)

When Symptoms Appear: 2-7 days after being infected.

Symptoms: females—thick, yellow or white discharge, burning with urination or bowel movement, and cramps in lower abdomen; males—discharge/drip from penis, burning with urination, difficulty having or a strong urge to have a bowel movement, discomfort or pain with bowel movement, and bloody stools.

How Contracted: vaginal, oral or anal intercourse.

Cure: antibiotics are used for treatment; some people have built up a resistance to penicillin which can make this STD hard to treat; partner must also be treated.

What Can Happen If Not Treated Or Cured: sterility; infections that can damage joints and heart tissue; blindness in newborns from vaginal delivery; PID (pelvic inflammatory disease).

STD: Hepatitis B

When Symptoms Appear: 6 weeks to 6 months after being infected.

Symptoms: flu-like symptoms including sore muscles or joints, sore throat, fever, nausea, vomiting, fatigue; pale stools and dark urine occur when liver is infected; skin and whites of eyes develop a yellow tone.

How Contracted: sharing needles; vaginal, oral or anal intercourse; baby born to infected mother; sharing blood/body fluids; blood transfusions; disease most contagious when there are no symptoms.

Cure: blood test is needed for diagnosis; bed rest is only treatment; every child, during or before adolescence, should have the Hepatitis B vaccine.

What Can Happen If Not Treated Or Cured: cancer; liver disease; death.

STD: Hepatitis C

When Symptoms Appear: 2 weeks to 6 months after exposure (symptoms most often appear between 6-9 weeks).

Symptoms: flu-like symptoms, although most people never show any signs at all.

How Contracted: vaginal, anal or oral intercourse; sharing blood through infected needles.

Cure: rest.

What Can Happen if Not Treated Or Cured: liver disease.

STD: Herpes

When Symptoms Appear: 2-10 days after being infected and lasting 2-3 weeks.

Symptoms: small painful blisters on sex organs or mouth; tingling before blisters appear; burning or painful urination.

How Contracted: direct contact with blisters or area of tingling; vaginal, oral or rectal contact; someone can be contagious for a few days before sores actually appear.

Treatment: there is no cure for herpes; prescription medication can only ease and control the symptoms that may appear often, every once-in-a-while or never again; blisters may come back when the person is tired, sick or stressed.

What Can Happen If Not Treated: cervical cancer; death or brain damage may occur in infants infected at birth through a vaginal delivery.

STD: Pelvic Inflammatory Disease (PID)

When Symptoms Appear: may have symptoms as soon as the first menstrual period after being infected.

Symptoms: lower abdominal pain; fever; discharge or bleeding from the vagina; nausea, vomiting and diarrhea.

How Contracted: infection from other STDs like gonorrhea or chlamydia has spread to uterus and fallopian tubes (where a fertilized egg passes to the uterus).

Cure: antibiotics are used for treatment.

What Can Happen if Not Treated Or Cured: may cause scarring of fallopian tubes which can affect ability to have children or can result in miscarriage.

STD: Pubic Lice (Crabs/Scabies)

When Symptoms Appear: symptoms may appear as soon as 24 hours after exposure.

Symptoms: small, nearly invisible insects found in the hair on body, face and/or genitals; intense itching or bluish spots where lice have bitten.

How Contracted: may or may not be transmitted sexually (can also occur from sharing clothes, bed sheets, towels and through contact with a contaminated toilet seat (although this rarely happens because the lice don't live very long on a toilet seat).

Cure: must see a health care professional for information on different types of over-the-counter and prescriptions lotions or powders; partner must also be treated.

What Can Happen If Not Treated Or Cured: lice won't go away without treatment; itching will only get worse, and insects will spread to other parts of the body.

STD: Syphilis

When Symptoms Appear: 1st stage, 1-12 weeks; 2nd stage, 2-12 weeks; 3rd stage, 3 years or more.

Symptoms: 1st stage: painless sores (called chancres) on genitals or mouth; 2nd stage: low fever, rash, spotty hair loss, sore throat, swollen glands; 3rd stage: no obvious signs; symptoms can disappear without treatment, but infection remains.

How Contracted: direct contact (sexually or not) with infectious sores, rashes or fluid from sores (can also be spread by contact with dirty towels, sheets and clothing).

Cure: blood test needed for diagnosis; antibiotics are used for treatment; symptoms may disappear without treatment, but not the disease itself; partner must also be treated.

What Can Happen If Not Treated Or Cured: death; heart disease; spinal cord or brain damage; blindness; damage to skin, bones, eyes, teeth and blood vessels; ulcers on the skin and internal organs; arthritis; loss of feeling in arms and legs; liver disease in infants.

STD: Trichomoniasis

When Symptoms Appear: 1-4 weeks after being infected.

Symptoms: females—heavy, frothy discharge from vagina with intense itching and burning; males—clear discharge with itching after urination.

How Contracted: direct contact with infected area with or without sexual contact (may contract the disease by sharing dirty towels, sheets or clothing).

Cure: antibiotics are used for treatment.

What Can Happen If Not Treated Or Cured: gland infection.

STD: Venereal Warts (Condyloma, Human Papillomavirus-HPV, Genital Warts)

When Symptoms Appear: 3 months to several years after being infected.

Symptoms: irritation; itching; wart growths with cauliflower-like tops on genitals, anus, cervix or throat.

How Contracted: easily caught through direct contact with warts; the virus can also be spread whether warts are present or not; a wart on someone's hand cannot cause genital warts.

Treatment: there is no cure for the virus; genital warts can be removed by a doctor or other health professional by freezing or burning them off or with surgery or lasers; warts grow back in 30% of people who have been treated; partner should also be treated.

What Can Happen If Not Treated: cancer of cervix, vagina or penis.

Find Out For Sure . . . Guessing Can Be Dangerous

If found and treated early, some STDs can be controlled or cured by medication. It's important to catch them before they affect your chances of having children, getting cancer or even dying. Guessing can be dangerous. If you think you have an STD, see a health professional immediately.

STD germs are hard to kill. You must do exactly what your doctor or other health professional tells you. Be sure to use all of your medicine. Douching does not work and may cause the infection to spread. If the symptoms disappear without treatment, it doesn't mean the infection is gone.

You also must tell your sexual partner(s). If they aren't treated, they can spread the STD and might even give it to you again.

Not every weird discharge, pain or sore means you

have an STD. Some of the same symptoms are common with other infections that have nothing at all to do with sex. Don't panic—but be sure to have it checked out by a health professional.

What You Don't Know Can Kill You

STD: AIDS (HIV)

AIDS deserves a little more consideration on your part because it has no age limit—and no mercy. It doesn't matter if you're male, female, black, white, rich, poor, gay or straight. You can get AIDS and die.

Approximately 1 million Americans are infected with HIV—about 1 in every 250 people. And teenage AIDS cases are on the rise. In fact, many people in their twenties who are now being diagnosed with AIDS caught the virus when they were kids.

The Human Immunodeficiency Virus (HIV) is the cause of AIDS. A virus is a small germ that can cause disease. AIDS, or Acquired Immunodeficiency Syndrome, is the result of a long process that begins with HIV infection. AIDS can destroy the body's immune system making it unable to fight off even small infections. The virus can also attack the nervous system, causing seizures, memory loss and mental disorders. Everyone who gets AIDS dies. There is no cure.

How Could I Get AIDS?

You can get AIDS by having sex (even once) with someone who has the virus. During sex, the virus contained in blood, semen or other body fluids can enter your body. You can get AIDS by body piercing, tattooing or by shooting drugs or steroids with a needle, syringe or other equipment that still has traces of blood from an infected person on it (you may not be able to see the blood with the naked eye). Girls can pass the virus on to their babies during pregnancy and birth and when breast-feeding. People also have been infected by receiving blood transfusions. (Today this risk is small because donors are screened and their blood tested for the AIDS antibody before use.)

AIDS is not caused by mosquitoes, casual contact such as holding hands or drinking from the same glass, or using the same toilet. You also don't have to worry about getting it from your doctor, dentist or the waitperson at a restaurant.

There is a small risk of getting AIDS through deep, wet french kissing because cuts and sores in the mouth may provide a way for HIV to enter the bloodstream. Most scientists agree, however, it would take a lot of saliva to pass the virus this way.

People can be infected with HIV for up to ten years or more without symptoms before progressing to AIDS. Once symptoms appear they may include fatigue, fever, loss of appetite and weight, swollen glands, white spots or un-usual blemishes in the mouth, night sweats, pneumo-nia, skin cancer and diarrhea. For those who engage in risky behavior, an HIV antibody test can determine if there has been exposure to the virus.

How Can I Be Sure I Don't Have HIV/AIDS?

The only way you can find out if you have HIV is by hav-ing a blood test. These tests look for antibodies to the virus (antibodies help fight infection and disease). You can be tested—in private—by a doctor or at a local health department, family planning clinic or other state testing site. In most places, you use a number to find out your results, so no one has to know your real name or where you live.

A positive test means you have been infected with HIV and can give it to other people. It doesn't necessar-ily mean you have full-blown AIDS. You should protect yourself and others from further infection, see a doctor for treatment, eat well, exercise and stay healthy. Most importantly, seek counseling from a professional.

A negative test means no antibodies have been found. You may not be infected at all (hopefully!), or your body may not have started fighting the infection yet. (Most people produce antibodies 2-8 weeks after being infected. Some will not produce them for 6 months. A few may never.) A negative test does not mean you can't or won't get the disease. Think about it! Protect yourself!

Protecting Yourself

To reduce your risk of getting an STD, you and your partner must practice safer sex:

- Wait to have sex. Abstinence is the only SAFE sex.

- Give yourself more time to be sure you are ready to have sex.

- Limit your number of sexual partners to one (none is safest).

- Ask your partner about his or her past sexual partners. When you have sex, you're not only having it with each other but every other partner that has come before you.

- Ask your partner about his or her needle and drug use, past history of STDs and whether they had a blood transfusion before1985 (before blood was screened for HIV).

- Ask them if they've been tested for STDs or HIV and to see the results.

- Take charge. Don't rely on someone else to use protection or to use it the right way. Partners may not know they're infected or may not tell the truth about it.

- Avoid sexual contact with someone who has symptoms of STDs. (Yet don't shy away or avoid someone with an STD or HIV/AIDS. Your friendship may be their only light in what could be a very dark future.)

- Don't drink alcohol or do drugs—they can lead you to do things you wouldn't do drug-free and put you at risk.

- Don't shoot drugs/steroids or share equipment to shoot drugs.

- Avoid sharing razors or equipment used for tattooing and body piercing.

- Use a new, latex condom and a contraceptive spermicide every time before and during vaginal, oral or anal sex.

- Have regular health checkups.

- Have an HIV (AIDS) antibody test if your behaviors place you at risk and ask your partner to do the same (if he or she refuses, you should say "no" to sex).

- Keep using protection long after you've decided your partner is "safe."

- Repeat over and over to yourself: "A few minutes of pleasure isn't worth dying for."

Check It Out

This information is intended to inform, not scare you. The thing to remember with AIDS—and all other STDs—is to be careful and think before you act.

The same people who can give you reliable information about birth control are there to help you if you think you might have a sexually transmitted disease. Doctors and other qualified health professionals at local health departments, hospitals and clinics offer confidential and anonymous counseling and testing. Anonymous means they don't ask who you are. Confidential means, in most cases, the information will not be shared with anyone else without your permission.

You could make yourself sick just worrying about STDs, and even sicker if fear keeps you from getting diagnosed and treated. Learn the facts. Act safely and responsibly. Check things out if you're worried. Guessing can be dangerous. Besides, life and love aren't any fun if you're sick, dying or dead.

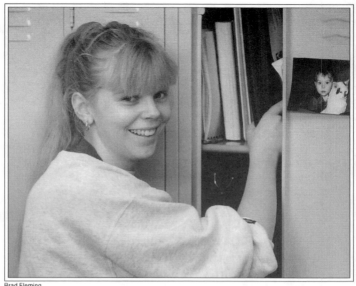

Brad Fleming

4

Joy

Joy has big plans for herself. She's working hard to keep a 3.8 grade average in school. She's looking ahead to college because she hopes to be a photojournalist. She wants to get married and have children.

There's only one thing Joy didn't plan on: getting pregnant at sixteen.

I was stupid. I didn't think I would get pregnant. I'd been having unprotected sex for a long time, so I wasn't really worried about it.

Besides, I thought I could deal with it if it happened. I was wrong.

When I look back I guess I didn't like myself much. I started drinking when I was 10, dropped acid at 11 and began having unprotected sex at 13. I thought having sex was a way to get people to like you. That is completely wrong. You lose their respect.

I lost a lot of friends. They either didn't approve or they dropped me because I couldn't party with them anymore. My boyfriend went to prison when I was eight months pregnant. My parents were disappointed, especially my dad. I had always been his little girl. It was a very lonely time.

My son Forrest is 16 months old now. We live on $351 a month from ADC (Aid to Dependent Children). I pay my mom $120 a month for child care and room and board. We just scrape by.

The whole thing has made me grow up fast. Before I had the baby I dropped out of school. I didn't want to go and look big and pregnant.

Once I gave birth to my son, I knew that in order to keep my life on track I had to graduate. An alternative school program made that possible. I learned a lot there. They offered parenting and childbirth classes, academic courses and day care.

Without the program, I couldn't finish school, go to college or get a good job. I also received a lot of support and encouragement along the way. The people there taught me to value myself. They helped me see myself as a winner who could do anything if I put my mind to it.

If Only...

If only Joy had known that most pregnancies happen within six months of the first unprotected intercourse.

If only she had known how lonely life was going to be. That by the time the blood test comes back positive, most teenage fathers are long gone. That few teenage mothers marry the father and of those who do, nearly 60% (60 out of every 100) end up divorced.

If only she had known that between diapers, medical bills, clothes, housing and food, it costs nearly $200,000 to raise a child to the age of 18. That's why most teenage parents live in poverty.

If only Joy knew then what she knows now.

Hey Guys, This Isn't Just A "Chick Thing"

If you're having unprotected sex with a girl, you better start saving your money now. You're going to be responsible for some of that $200,000 bill to raise your child.

Some states are hard on deadbeat dads. If you don't keep up with child support, you may lose part of your paycheck at work and any tax refunds you might be getting. You may find credit collectors all over your back and even end up in jail. If you don't have a job and can't pay support, your parents may have to. (That will make them really happy!?!)

There's more to all this than just money. If you think getting a girl pregnant makes you more of a man, you may be in for a surprise. What you really may be is a man without a future—with less hanging time with friends, less education, a low paying job and a lot more bills to pay. Most importantly, you and your child will pay for your selfishness and carelessness for the rest of your lives. Just remember, any guy can get a girl pregnant. But it's not every guy who is smart enough to use protection and wait to have kids. If your girl does get pregnant, stick by her. Be a *real* man.

Do More Than Think. . .Find Out For Sure

If you think you may be pregnant, find out for sure. This problem will not go away on its own. Missing a period, tender breasts, being sick to your stomach (morning sickness) and feeling tired all the time are just a few of the signs of pregnancy.

You can start with a home pregnancy test from the drugstore, but don't rely on the results one hundred percent. The best way to be sure is by having a confidential blood test at a clinic or doctor's office. A blood test cannot only confirm pregnancy but also tell you how far along you are.

Take Your Time

Once you find out for sure, DON'T DO ANYTHING...at least for awhile. Take your time. Catch your breath. Cry until you work through your panic. A few days of deep thinking is not going to make or break the situation.

Find Out All Your Options

Look at both the risks and benefits. Talk it over with your partner, your parents, and school and family planning counselors. Don't try to work this problem out on your own.

When you tell people, expect a lot of different reactions. Your boyfriend may be shocked, happy, scared or all three. He may stay with you or disappear forever. Your friends will freak out and either dump you or support you. Your parents may blow up at you or cry. You're still their baby. They love you and see all of their hopes and dreams going up in smoke.

Your choices are not simple ones. So, spend a great deal of time thinking everything through before deciding what to do, because for the rest of your life, you'll wonder whether you did the right thing.

Take Care Of Yourself

You should see a doctor or midwife (another health professional who helps mothers with pregnancy and childhood) on a regular basis. Without good prenatal care, both you and your baby face a greater risk of illness and death.

Don't worry about asking too many questions. There's a lot you need to know. You have to eat the right foods, take vitamins made especially for pregnant women, and exercise safely. You may want to have an HIV test. There are things that can be done to protect your baby from the virus before he's ever born.

You must also stop smoking or taking illegal drugs or medicines that could harm or kill you and the baby. For each pull on a cigarette, swig of beer or sniff of coke you take, your baby takes one, too. Alcohol, cigarettes and drugs can hurt your unborn baby in ways that can't be fixed. He can be born addicted to drugs, deformed, retarded or, worse, dead at birth.

You, too, put yourself at risk of miscarriage, suffering through a dangerous and painful labor and infertility (never being able to have another child). You could also lose your new baby to foster care if you are deemed an unfit mother.

Your doctor is the best person to tell you what to expect while you're pregnant and teach you how to stay healthy. Follow his suggestions and give you and your baby a good start.

Stay In School

If going back to high school isn't possible, check out alternative education programs. These programs offer high school classes, pre-baby and after-baby education and care, parenting classes and group, individual and career counseling. Both your future and the baby's may depend on you sticking with school.

Protect Yourself From Another Pregnancy

You know that nearly one million teenage girls get pregnant every year. Believe it or not, at least one in every five of them will get pregnant again within a year. Lightening can strike twice. Don't make the same mistake.

Protect yourself or choose to be a virgin for the second time.

What Kind Of Life Is This For A Child? For You?

You may wish you had a baby. Someone to love and care for. You just know you'd be a good parent. But understand that you are probably dooming yourself, as well as your child, to a hard, hard life

Parenting is not all sweetness and light. Starting with that first grueling labor pain, your baby is going to demand your full attention. Just consider that the last good night's sleep you'll ever have is the night you conceive. You'll be dragged out of bed every 2-3 hours at night for a feeding. You'll carry diapers, wipes, formula, food, blankets and an extra change of clothing—everywhere you go—even to the bathroom. You will rarely do anything by or for yourself again, at least until that child is grown and on his own. Even then, you'll still be a mother with all of the legal, physical and emotional responsibilities that go with the job.

Your child may be destined to a life without enough money, the right care or a good education. Most kids born to teenage parents drop out of school; wind up in juvenile hall, foster care or prison; don't have jobs; and have children when they're still children. And so the cycle repeats itself.

The greatest way to show love for yourself and a child is by not getting pregnant until you're older and better prepared. If you want a future for yourself, use your hopes and dreams as birth control.

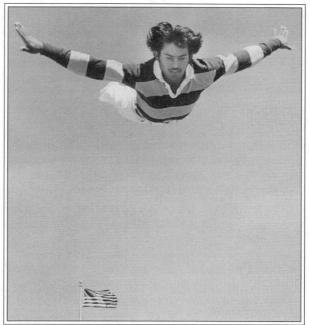
Brad Fleming

5

Body Talk

The extent to which we love ourselves determines whether we eat right, get enough sleep, don't smoke, wear seat belts, exercise and so on. Each of these choices is a statement of how much we care about living.

BERNIE S. SIEGEL, M.D.

87

Before you sit down for that next meal, tear open that candy wrapper or push the button on that pop machine, consider this:

- The effect of caffeine on your body doesn't reach its peak until 2 to 4 hours after you drink it. You may even be able to still feel its effect after 7 hours.

- Most non-diet sodas contain 8 to 12 teaspoons of sugar in a 12 ounce can.

- Eating 8 ounces of potato chips is like adding 12 to 20 teaspoons of vegetable oil and a teaspoon of salt to an 8 ounce baked potato - as much fat and sodium as most people should eat in a day.

- Snacking on 2 ounces of chocolate is the same as eating 4 teaspoons of butter or oil and 10 teaspoons of sugar.

The Food Pyramid

When you read and hear about the food pyramid, pay attention. It's not just another thing to remember for health class.

Eating right can really make a difference in how you look and feel. How much energy you have. The mood you're in. Your weight, skin, hair and smile.

Foods like milk, fruits, vegetables and grains (pasta, cereal and bread) work together in your body. If you only eat from a few food groups, you won't get all the vitamins, minerals and nutrients your body needs. And at your age, extra nutrients may be necessary to keep up with the rate you're growing.

Carbohydrates are to your body what gas is to a car. They fuel the body and give you energy. A certain amount of fat in your diet helps keep your skin in good condition and your hair shiny. Protein provides the building materials for growth and the care and repair of the body's cells. Vitamins, minerals and iron help keep your bones and teeth strong and give your body the strength to heal injuries and fight infection. Depending upon how active you are, you may need to eat 2,000-4,000 calories a day.

Eating a balanced diet and snacking only once in a while are also the best ways to keep your teeth forever and your smile beautiful. Hard candies, suckers and "jelly" candies dissolve slowly and coat your teeth with sugar. Then—you guessed it—tooth decay.

Brush at least twice a day or after every meal (especially if you have braces) with a soft brush, paying special attention to the line where your teeth and gums meet. Floss daily. Even though it's a pain to get started on a flossing routine, once you do, you'll never stop. Visiting a dentist every six months to have your teeth cleaned is also important for keeping those "choppers" for a lifetime.

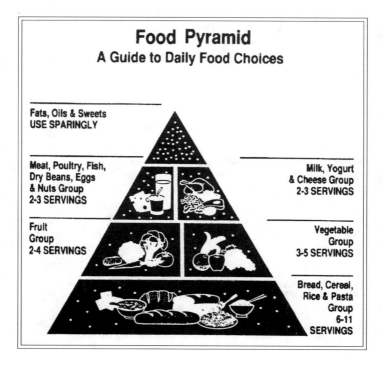

Food Pyramid
A Guide to Daily Food Choices

Fats, Oils & Sweets
USE SPARINGLY

Meat, Poultry, Fish,
Dry Beans, Eggs
& Nuts Group
2-3 SERVINGS

Milk, Yogurt
& Cheese Group
2-3 SERVINGS

Fruit
Group
2-4 SERVINGS

Vegetable
Group
3-5 SERVINGS

Bread, Cereal,
Rice & Pasta
Group
6-11
SERVINGS

Your One And Only Body

How bad is skipping a meal, like breakfast?

Just like a car needs gas to keep it going, you need food to keep going. If you skip breakfast, your body and brain haven't been fueled since dinner the night before and are likely to give out right in the middle of traffic. It's a proven fact: people are not as alert and are more irritable and tired when their bodies don't have enough fuel.

Will skipping meals help with weight loss?

Most people skip a meal only to make up for it later in the day. So, for dieting, skipping stinks. Eating healthy, low-fat meals from the food pyramid, watching calories and exercising often are the best ways to lose weight.

If I usually eat a good diet, is it okay to sometimes chow down on fast foods?

It's fast and cheap. What more could you want from fast food? How about a little less fat, calories and so-dium.

How often you should eat fast foods depends on how active you are. How often do you play ball, go rollerblading, skiing, swimming or go for a walk?

Once a week is okay if you don't have a weight prob-lem, and you're very active. But eating fast foods on a regular basis may cost you in the long run.

Some fast foods are high in calories, fat and sodium. Health experts believe too much sodium and fat causes high blood pressure, obesity, heart disease and cancer. If you sit down and eat a cheeseburger, fries, chocolate shake and dessert, you have already had more calories, fat and sodium than you need in one entire day!

You don't have to avoid these foods like the plague, you just can't overdo it. If you had a fast food frenzy at lunch, eat a healthy, low-calorie, low-fat dinner. Watch how much you eat on the basis of one whole day.

When you go to your favorite fast food joint, order a broiled hamburger with mustard, lettuce and pickles. Broiled chicken sandwiches are also good, as are turkey sandwiches (hold the mayonnaise) and salad (go easy on the dressing and skip the bacon bits).

What's the big deal about fat?

The best diet is not one totally without fat. In fact, it's important to have a certain amount of fat for healthy skin and hair. Some fat is also needed for proper growth and the absorption of certain vitamins into your system.

What if I just become a vegetarian?

There are different types of vegetarians. Some don't eat red meat but do include chicken and fish in their diet. Others don't eat any kind of animal or fish (including eggs and milk products) and stick with vegetables and grains only. If you're thinking about doing this, talk to someone who knows a lot about nutrition. Red meat, for example, supplies a lot of calcium, iron, zinc and protein. Without it, your body and looks could suffer. You'll need to make up for the loss in the other things you eat, and a nutrition expert can tell you how.

Do diet drinks, diet pills and fad diets really work?

You've heard the commercials and seen the ads. The message these days is: "thin is in." You're in for trouble if you take this advice too seriously.

First of all, the "skin and bones" look is no longer in. Today's look is healthy and athletic. Even top models are into the balanced diet, regular exercise routine. Many of them have found out the hard way that fad dieting is the worst way to lose weight.

When you use pills and drinks to curb your appetite, your body learns to live on fewer calories than it did before. Once you start eating normally again, your weight will come back fast. Besides, when you starve yourself, you slow down your metabolism. Yet, you need a high metabolism to burn fat, so you really end up defeating the purpose.

Losing weight isn't about going on a diet; it's about changing the way you live. There's nothing noble about being able to go for one whole day on only a handful of crackers. Anyone can do that. You'll feel greater pride if you learn which foods and nutrients you need, cut the fat and exercise. After all, if you're not healthy after losing weight, what good does it do you?

Strict dieting is especially harmful for teenage girls. They often begin weighing themselves constantly and tie their self-image to the numbers on the scale. Then dieting and food become all the person thinks about, leading to depression and eating disorders.

Eating Disorders

Eight million Americans, especially teenage girls (though guys can have them, too) between the ages of 13 and 20, suffer from eating disorders...150,000 die each year. Eating disorders have more to do with a person's emotions than her body.

Anorexia nervosa, sometimes called the "disease of denial," often affects girls who have low self-esteem, are perfectionists, high achievers and control freaks. Anorexics, who may be underweight to begin with, starve themselves because they feel fat and are afraid of gaining weight. But the problem isn't food. Usually, a person with eating disorders is worried or upset over other things happening in their lives.

In the fifth grade, I happened to be the one everybody picked on. I didn't know why, and I finally decided it was because I was fat. If I lost a couple of pounds, they might like me. I mean, if they didn't like me, why should I like me?

KATIE, 15

Signs of Trouble: Anorexia Nervosa
A person suffering from anorexia nervosa shows signs of:
- extreme weight loss
- eating less
- denying hunger

- excessive exercise
- extreme fear of being fat
- rigid self-control

I just wanted everything to be perfect. So I thought I'd lose a few pounds. It got to where I would just eat a handful of crackers all day. I would lie to my parents and tell them I'd eaten. I quit sitting with my friends because they were always asking me why I wasn't having something. I finally collapsed.

KARA, 16

People with bulimia binge, meaning they eat large amounts of food in a short period of time. Then they get rid of it—or "purge"—by vomiting, exercising like crazy, taking laxatives or fasting (not eating for a time). In private, bulimics may go on marathon eating sprees, wolfing down thousands of calories in a day.

This so-called "disease of secrecy" is a vicious cycle. Binging leads to guilt and fear of weight gain which leads to purging which brings on guilt and disgust which leads to starvation which is followed by another binge session.

Signs of Trouble: Bulimia
A person with bulimia:
- layers their clothes to hide weight loss
- has mood swings
- makes excuses to go to the bathroom
- leaves the bathroom with the smell of vomit
- buys and eats a lot of food
- makes excuses not to eat with others
- thinks constantly about weight and body image
- isolates herself from friends and family
- has suicidal feelings

I got to the point where I was taking 60 laxatives and throwing up 6 times every day. And that was on top of 3-4 hours of exercise. My biggest fear was someone finding out and thinking I was a freak.

ANNE, 17

Your Body Can't Take It

At first, binging and purging or starvation offers relief from the stressful feelings of poor self-esteem and depression. It makes the girl feel more in control of her life. Unfortunately, the bad feelings become worse. The person often separates herself from family and friends which only leads to a deeper sense of depression and helplessness.

Many bulimics and anorexics don't even realize how serious the problem is until they start having physical problems. They think this is a great way to keep their weight and life in control. But not eating or repeated vomiting can be very, very dangerous. Eating disorders have sent many people to the hospital with serious damage to their heart, liver and kidneys.   One in ten anorexics die.

Others may suffer from:
- light-headedness, sweating and shaking
- blood disorders and loss of menstrual cycle
- abnormal heart beat and the shrinking of the heart muscle leading to a heart attack
- the growth of fine hair on the face, shoulders, back and arms
- stomach problems
- fatigue, no energy
- deformed bone growth and osteoporosis (weakening of the bones which leads to easy fractures).

Forced vomiting with bulimia can tear the esophagus (swallowing tube) and cause bleeding of the stomach or intestines and colon disorders.

Laxatives do more to cause stomach pain, constipation and diarrhea than they do to reduce calories. Stomach acids from vomiting also destroy tooth enamel causing severe tooth decay, discoloration and gum damage.

The greatest danger to the bulimic is that the problem can be kept secret for a long time. A girl can go several years without anyone being the wiser, and therefore, without treatment.

It's been a long struggle, but I'm a different person today. My advice to anyone who thinks they have an eating disorder is: you can't fix it on your own. You need people who can help you focus on what's good in your life.

KARA, 20

Treating bulimia and anorexia requires both a body and mind approach. A physical exam will help to determine if damage has been done to internal organs. Individual counseling, behavior and nutrition modification (learning to eat and think about food differently), family therapy and support groups are also used to stop the cycle. Little by little, the bulimic or anorexic learns to rely on others for help instead of food.

Now that I've started eating, I have more friends. My grades are up. I'm more active. I sing, play the piano and take tennis lessons. I'm just happier. My attitude has changed. I smile now, that's the big difference.

LIZ, 17

How can I help a friend who has an eating disorder?

- Let the person know you're worried, that you care, and most importantly, that you want to help.

- Don't talk about food or how the person looks. Try talking about anything but food. Ask her how she feels. Try to find out what's really bothering her.

- Don't tell the person how terribly thin she is. That

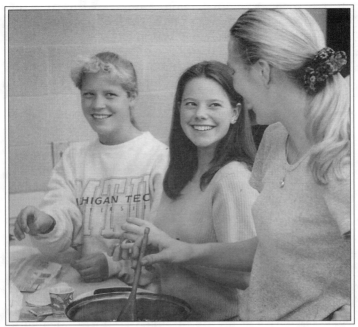

Brad Fleming

will encourage her. She thinks the thinner she is the better.

- Don't say how much better they look if they start gaining weight. They'll just think they're getting fat again.

- Try to get her to talk with a parent, counselor, doctor or someone who's opinion she values. At some point, you may need to tell someone else who can step in and help.

I don't have an eating disorder, but I really do have a major problem with my weight? What do I do?

Don't let the bathroom scales tell you you're overweight. Weighing a lot and being obese are two very different things. Muscle weighs twice as much as fat. So, you may weigh heavy for your size but have more muscle and less fat (which is good) than somebody who weighs less than you. A few people who are really obese have medical problems that affect their ability to lose weight. Most of the time though, obesity is caused by a lack of exercise and poor eating habits like:

- eating fast and on the run
- skipping breakfast and lunch and chowing down on dinner
- eating a lot of junk food
- turning to food when depressed or upset

The longer a child is truly overweight, the more likely they'll be that way as adults. Along with their weight, they may suffer from high blood pressure, heart disease, some types of cancer, stroke, diabetes and growth problems. Some people also become very lonely and depressed. They hide away because they're embarrassed to be seen, which only makes it harder to fight the weight.

If you want to lose weight:

- motivate yourself—put your mind to it and do it
- go and see a doctor for some advice and a checkup
- get your whole family involved in exercising and eating right
- join a support group or get counseling to keep you going and boost your self-confidence

How often should I see a doctor for a checkup?

You may live longer and healthier with regular checkups. So, it's a good idea to visit your family doctor or other health professional at least once a year. Health care providers like to see you regularly to chart height and weight and to watch for any growth problems. Your doctor may also be able to detect problems early when they are more easily treated and cured.

Young women have added health concerns. Once menstruation begins, breast exams, pelvic exams and PAP tests become important, as well as screening for sexually

Recommended* Annual Physical Examinations

Medical History
Height and Weight
Blood Pressure
Urinalysis
Developmental Assessment
Behavioral Assessment

HEALTH SCREENINGS	RECOMMENDED AGE
Pelvic (Females)	Every year at 18
PAP Smear (Females)	Every year at 18 or when sexually active
Breast Exam (Females)	Every year at 18
Breast Self Exam	Monthly at 18
Testicular Exam (Males)	Every year
Self Testicular Exam	Monthly starting at 15
Hearing Test	As needed
Vision Test	Yearly
Tuberculin Skin Test	Yearly with high risk
Anemia Screening	As needed
Serum Cholesterol	As needed
Mumps, Measles, Rubella Booster	Preschool or at 13 years
Tetanus/Diphtheria	15 years and every 10 years
Sexually Transmitted Disease Screening	As needed
Dental Health Exam & Cleaning	Every 6 months
Hepatitis B	Newborn or before or during adolescence

*Depending on past medical and immunization history.

transmitted diseases if she is sexually active (guys should also be screened if sexually active).

Are there things I can check myself?

Yes. You can and should take charge of your own health. In fact, many problems are first detected through self-exams.

Guys: do a simple, 3-minute exam of your testicles every month. It may seem stupid, but cancer of the testes—the male reproductive glands—is one of the most common cancers in men ages 15-34. If testicular cancer is found early, it can often be cured.

Girls: check your breasts for lumps every month starting at age 18. This simple act could not only save your breast, but your life. Most breast lumps are found by women themselves, and many aren't cancerous. Lumps that are a sign of cancer can be more easily treated and cured if found early. Even though it may seem uncomfortable at first, be safe and be sure by spending only 15 minutes a month examining your breasts.

Your doctor and other qualified health professionals can teach you these self-examination techniques. The American Cancer Society also has "how to" brochures.

How important is exercise?

If you sit around all day, you may be facing obesity, heart disease and other lifelong problems. So, if you aren't already exercising, start now! Join a sports team or aerobics group. If you like to go solo, walk! It's cheap and easy!

When you run, play ball, lift weights, or whatever, your body produces endorphins which give you a natural high and a feeling of strength and well-being.

By exercising regularly, you can:
- improve your heart's ability to pump blood
- prevent heart disease
- lower high blood pressure
- gain stronger muscles

- be more flexible
- control your weight
- control stress
- prevent injury
- improve self-image and self-confidence
- have a better looking body

How much is enough?

If you want to improve the condition of your heart and lungs, you have to get your heart and breathing rates up there. The American College of Sports Medicine suggests aerobic exercise like playing basketball, rollerblading, skiing, hiking, running, jumping rope, rowing, and cycling at least 15 to 60 minutes, 3-5 times a week. Even walking at a solid pace just 30 minutes a day can improve the state of your heart, keep your weight in check and keep your spirits up.

How much is too much?

Using the same muscles over and over again can result in sprains, strains and stress fractures. All of your muscles need to rest sometime. Cross-training, or alternating exercise plans, allows you to work out different muscles on different days. Run one day, lift weights the next. It's one of the best ways to reach total body fitness.

I like the way I look with a tan. Why should I worry about baking under the sun?

Doctors and scientists are learning more and more about the damaging rays of the sun. There are two types of rays that reach from the sun. The short beta or UVB rays damage the outer layers of the skin known as the epidermis. This damage can result in wrinkles, premature aging and skin cancer.

The second type of ray, the long alpha or UVA rays, reach farther down than the UVB rays to the dermis or base layer of the skin. Because they reach so deep, UVA rays cause more serious harm including aging, sagging, skin cancer, and possibly, allergic reactions. The rays can also break down the tissue of elastin which supports the skin. You end up with skin that looks like old alligator hide. Maybe you look good with a tan now, but wait until you hit 40 and look 60.

According to the American Cancer Society, more than 600,000 new cases of skin cancer are reported every year. It's the most common form of cancer. It's also one of the easiest to cure when it's found and treated early. Better still, you can prevent skin cancer altogether.

How can I protect myself?

The sun's rays are just as harmful in the winter as in the summer. That's why you need to protect yourself all year long. The damage done by UVA and UVB rays also builds up year after year.

To take care of your skin, put on sunscreen 30 minutes before going out into the sun. Look for suntan lotions that block both UVA and UVB rays, with at least an SPF of 15. The SPF (sun protection factor) of a lotion is a way of measuring it's ability to screen out the UVB rays of the sun. The SPF number tells you how long you can stay out in the sun and still be protected.

If your lotion says "SPF 15," for example, you should be able to stay out in the sun and be protected 15 times longer than without the lotion. Check the bottle for directions on how often you need to reapply the lotion. Some last as long as 8 hours. Others should be reapplied after swimming or perspiring, or every two hours for best protection.

Watch out! The sun is strongest between 11 a.m. and 2 p.m., and neither clouds nor water will protect you from its far-reaching rays.

Are tanning booths any safer than the sun?

Many of us want to keep that "healthy glow" year-round; so we bake under the lights of a tanning booth. Before you do, consider the darker side. Using tanning booths or sunlamps may be as harmful as outdoor tanning. The risks include: skin cancer, premature aging, skin and eye burns, allergic reactions, cataracts (clouding of the eyes), reduced immunity (the body's ability to fight off infection), and blood vessel damage.

Like the sun, sunlamps and tanning booths give off both UVA and UVB rays. Some tanning salons may claim their sunlamps are safer than the sun, but both rays can be harmful. Because tanning booths allow you to tan year-round, they may actually be worse for you.

It's best not to tan, but if you decide to, in spite of the risks:

- Always use goggles that come with the tanning device and block out UV radiation. Make sure they fit snugly around your eyes and are not cracked. Don't rely on closing your eyes or using sunglasses or cotton wads.

- Learn your skin type and know how much sun it can handle.

- Be sure someone is nearby to help in an emergency.

Most doctors will advise you not to tan because one severe sunburn in childhood increases a person's lifetime risk of skin cancer by 70 percent.

Use common sense, whether you're under the sun or under the lamps. It's the best way to stay looking young and free of cancer.

How will I know if I have skin cancer?

You should be checked by a doctor if you have:

- a skin growth that increases in size and is tan, brown, black or multicolored

- a mole, birthmark, beauty mark or any brown spot that changes in size, thickness or feel, has an irregular shape or is bigger than the size of a pencil eraser

- a spot or sore that itches, hurts, bleeds and doesn't heal within three weeks.

I don't want to get a raging case of acne. Will I get it? If I do, how do I get rid of it?

Acne is really a deeper problem than you think. It

starts deep down below the surface of your skin where dead cells, dirt and oil mix together causing pores to form a plug and swell. Rumor has it that acne is caused by eating foods like chocolate, potato chips and ice cream. In fact, diet seems to have little effect on acne.

Acne can flare, however, by drinking and eating warm drinks, spicy foods or anything that makes the skin flush. Stress, nerves and drinking alcohol can also make matters worse. You may get acne if someone in your family has or had it. It may also show up on people with fair (light) skin or those who are nervous types or drink a lot of alcohol.

Most doctors recommend washing your face with a mild soap or alcohol-free cleansing product and patting dry. Scrubbing with harsh soap won't help and may even hurt. Avoid using oil-based skin products or ones which contain alcohol. Medications with cortisone, even non-prescription ones, don't work. If you notice the start of acne, take care of your skin and seek care early. Antibiotics or skin ointments, prescribed by your doctor, may help.

Although there is no cure for acne, don't wait to outgrow it. Waiting can result in scarring. Extreme cases may call for laser surgery to remove the scars. Counseling may also be needed if acne causes disfigurement.

To tattoo or not to tattoo?

People have been tattooing their bodies since the Ice Age. The first well-known person who sported a tattoo was Captain Cook, one of the first European explorers.

Today, tattooing is done not only for looks, but for medical reasons as well. Tattoo professionals often re-color scars from surgery or injury to match a person's normal skin tone.

Permanent tattooing is done by placing "pigment" color between the second and third layers of skin. The needle penetrates 40,000-50,000th of an inch, at a pulsing rate in and out of the skin at 360 times per second. A good tattooist uses new needles, disposable razor blades and small throwaway caps of color for onetime use only.

For the next ten days, using clean hands, apply a thin layer of antibacterial ointment to the open wound for proper healing. Any redness, swelling or lasting pain should be checked out by a health care professional.

Before having a tattoo, find an expert. Going to a nonprofessional places you at a greater risk of infection, disease or disfigurement. Find out if the tattoo "artist" has a practicing license or certificate. The best credentials come from the National Tattooing Association which is limited to only 1,000 approved members worldwide. A tattoo professional should also be a member of the Alliance of Professional Tattooists, which means they are attending classes and staying current on all infection and disease control issues. Scope out the methods they use, and watch them perform first. Find out how long the artist has been in the business, and ask for and check out references.

Tattoos last a lifetime. Before you get one, try the temporary ones. They last for several days and can be removed easily with cream or lotion. You can change them as often as your moods, and you won't be stuck with them forever. The long-term effects of permanent tattoos are still unknown, and they're difficult and painful to remove through repeated laser surgeries.

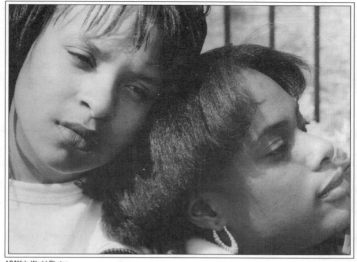

6

Melba

I started using drugs when I was 13. My family was in deep denial about anything I did. They just couldn't accept the fact that their daughter was doing these things. We weren't close. We didn't talk with each other. My father was an alcoholic, and his work took him away a lot. My mother focused more on that than what I was doing. Just growing up that way, I learned how to be manipulative and keep things secret.

Before I started using, I had certain expectations of myself. I thought I was pretty talented and somewhat intelligent. I even thought my initial decision to use was an intelligent one. I researched, and I knew what I was going to do. I knew what the side effects were. I wasn't going to be one of those kids who drank themselves through adolescence. But what really happened...

I ended up not caring about my studies, music and other things I was involved in. As my self-esteem started to plummet, I just dug myself a bigger hole. You can't get out. You can't stop. The more depressed you become, even about the little things you do, the more you want to use to cover them up.

I lost a lot of the friends who would have stood by me. I traded them in for people who were using—who are what they are. They're about the party, they're about the drunk, and that's all that they are. There's an assumed kind of maturity among people who party. They think, "We're older now. We can handle it." And that's really just a false front for a lot of lonely kids.

You spend all those years drinking and drugging, doing the party scene, and it puts you in all kinds of bad situations with guys, with violence, with AIDS. Now I worry about whether I'll come up with a disease.

I've spent my life in a four-year haze. That's time wasted. Time I could have spent doing all the fun things you're supposed to enjoy in life. You can't be 16, 17 or 18 years-old again. You can't get back the missed prom, the missed graduation.

I'm still struggling with my self esteem. I'm not in college, I'm not doing things kids my age are doing. I'm probably four years behind my friends because of the decisions I've made. Everyday I have to deal with the regret.

I lost some opportunities to go to a good school, to develop a good relationship with someone. A lot of my friends are getting married now. I am missing out on all that because my relationships were shallow and just based on partying and sex.

I'll never get back my virginity that was lost to alcohol and drugs. These are all personal and precious things that you can never get back. I'm never going to be innocent and naive and all the wonderful things you're supposed to be at that age.

Melba is 21 and has been in and out of recovery for drug addiction for the past seven years. With the help and support of many people, she's been clean now for more than a year.

Congratulations

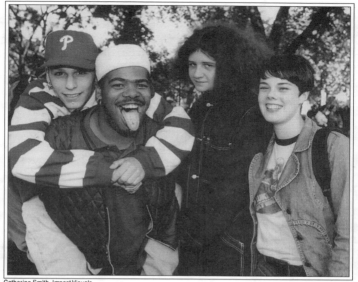

Catherine Smith, Impact Visuals

7

Point-blank

"But I only drink on weekends."

"I only smoke pot every once in a while."

"I only drink beer, not the hard stuff."

"My parents drink and nothing bad has happened to them."

You've heard the excuses. You may have used them before. Who are you kidding? If you think drugs are the ticket to fun and popularity, think again. When you decide to take drugs—whether it's alcohol, marijuana or cocaine—you're risking jail time, violence, heartache, even death.

You may also believe drugs take away your problems or make you more powerful against them. In fact, they make you less able to deal with them, until not only your problems eat you alive, but the drugs do, too. Very simply, the only thing wrong with drugs is...everything.

A Real Bad Habit

At first I just drank at parties. It made me feel more outgoing, looser, not so self-conscious, and it was fun. Pretty soon I was drinking a lot, just to keep up the good feeling. When I wasn't doing it, I noticed I wasn't feeling so great. So I drank more. Pretty soon I started first thing in the morning, all day long, and at night before I could fall asleep. I wanted to stop. But I felt like I couldn't. Somewhere in my mind I thought, 'This is killing me.'

MARK, 17

Drugs and alcohol are dangerous because they're addictive or habit-forming. Regular "users" develop a tolerance—a need to take more of the drug to get the same effect.

Certain drugs, including alcohol and nicotine, create physical dependence. With continued use, these drugs become part of your body's chemistry. When you stop taking them, the body can go through withdrawal. Depending upon the drug and how long it's been used, withdrawal can cause the shakes, nausea, vomiting, the sweats, violent behavior, depression, anxiety, scary hallucinations (seeing things that really aren't there), convulsions and sleeping problems.

If you become dependent on drugs, you go from taking drugs to feel good, to taking them to keep from feeling bad. Over time, drug use itself will increase the bad feelings and can leave you suicidal. In fact, more than half of all teenage suicides are drug-related.

Drugs Aren't Just A Quick High

Drugs can remain in the body long after you've stopped using them. For example, marijuana is fat-soluble, which means it seeks out and settles in the fatty tissues in our body such as the brain. As it builds in your system, the drug is slowly released over time and may affect the mind and body weeks or even months after drug use has stopped.

In truth, drug abuse of any kind—including nicotine, caffeine, alcohol, marijuana, inhalants and cocaine can lead to:

- problems with sexual desire and function (Your body has just started to grow sexually. Why would you want to mess that up now?)
- damage of your heart, respiratory (breathing) system and spinal cord
- mood disorders such as depression, anxiety or violent behaviors
- coma
- death
- babies that are born too early, addicted or still-born (dead at birth)

The Risks Aren't Worth It

A drug is a powerful thing. If you let it, it can control your life. I disagree with all the things drugs stand for and would never use them. I decided not to use them because I know what kind of person I want to be.

HEATHER, 15

You're an occasional user, not someone who's addicted. What's the big deal? Right?

Not too many addicts start out as constant users. You probably know people who have dropped out of school, gone to detention homes or jail, or given up all their hopes and dreams. The same thing could happen to you. Maybe the drug use has already started to become addictive, and you just haven't faced it.

You know the difference between right and wrong. Drugs are wrong—in the eyes of the law, the school, your family and even some of your friends. And if drugs are so appealing you would risk jail, being kicked out of school, being grounded or becoming addicted just to have them— even occasionally—it's pretty safe to say there's a problem.

It may be hard to believe these terrible things can happen to you. If and when you first try drugs and everything's cool, you'll think this is all just said to scare you. But you're not special when it comes to drugs. They can kill you just as easily as the next person. While you may ignore the advice, you can't deny the facts.

Alcohol: Point-blank

FACT: Alcohol is easy to get and doesn't cost much, which makes it the number one drug problem among kids today. Even though it is illegal in most states to drink under the age of 21, by their senior year of high school, almost all students will have tried alcoholic drinks. One in 20 kids will drink on a daily basis, and almost 4 out of 10 will consume 5 or more drinks in a row at least once every 2 weeks.

FACT: Beer, liquor, wine. Different names, different tastes, same amount of alcohol. As soon as the drink passes your taste buds, your body can't tell the difference. It reacts to any alcohol the same way and will have the same physical and emotional effects.

FACT: Alcohol goes directly into your bloodstream. In only a few minutes, it's circulating through your body. Yet, it takes three hours for your system to dispose of 1 1/2 ounces of liquor.

FACT: Alcohol is a downer. So, if you're drinking because you're stressed out, upset or bored, you can expect more of the same.

FACT: Drinking coffee or getting some fresh air will not sober you up. Only time can do that.

FACT: Drinking while on certain medications can make you a very sick person. Even medications like cold capsules, diet pills, acetaminophen (like Tylenol) and insulin can cause nausea, vomiting, convulsions, drowsiness and worse.

FACT: About half of all teenage deaths from drowning, fires, suicides and homicides are alcohol-related.

FACT: If you use alcohol now, when you're young, you're more likely to use it heavily and to have problems at school, at home and in your relationships with family and friends later in your life. You are also more likely to abuse other drugs, get into trouble with the law and be faced with an unplanned pregnancy.

FACT: Alcohol abuse can lead to premature aging, birth defects and fetal alcohol syndrome (FAS). Babies with FAS can suffer from retardation, low birth weight and deformities.

Heavy drinking for a long time can also make it tough to keep an erection during sex. Damage to sperm can lead to birth defects and an inability to have children.

Too much can cause high blood pressure, stomach disorders and damage to the brain and other major organs like the kidneys and liver. Cancers of the stomach, breast, colon, larynx (voice box) and esophagus (swallowing tube) can also be the results of long-term use. (And these effects can happen to females two times faster than males.)

FACT: Alcohol abuse costs the United States about $150 billion a year, and this price tag is expected to increase.

FACT: Puking is not very pretty and, with a hangover, you'll feel worse than death.

Drinking And Driving

FACT: Alcohol is the primary cause of car accidents involving teenage drivers and the leading cause of death among people ages 15-24.

FACT: The risk of being in an alcohol-related accident increases after only two drinks. With three drinks, the risk of a fatal crash jumps to 8 times as high compared with not drinking at all. With five drinks, that risk is 26 times higher.

FACT: If you are a passenger in a car, you have twice the chance of dying in an alcohol-related accident than the driver.

FACT: In more than half of all fatal accidents, drinking and/or drugs were involved.

FACT: More than 105,000 Americans die each year from injuries or diseases linked to alcohol—which works out to nearly 300 deaths each day.

The alcohol in a drink reaches the brain almost immediately. Whether you're behind the wheel of a car, a boat, a snowmobile or other vehicle, alcohol will have these effects:

- You can't concentrate as well and become tired.

- You don't see as well. Alcohol can cause double or multiple vision and blurring. Side vision may also be affected, making it difficult to see other vehicles approaching from the left or right.

- You have trouble making good and safe decisions. Alcohol dulls the area of the brain used to make decisions.

- You can't react as quickly. Drinking slows your reflexes. You won't be able to handle or control the car in dangerous situations.

You, Alcohol And The Law

Let's not cruise right by the fact that in many states it's against the law to drink until you're 21.

It doesn't do any good to throw those beer cans out of the car window. The law considers your body to be a container. If a breathalyzer test or a sample of your urine proves that you've been drinking—cans or no cans—you're a "minor in possession."

In some states, if you're at a party and alcohol is within your reach, you could be charged with possession —whether you've been drinking or not!

Know the laws in your state. Just a small amount of alcohol in your body, known as blood alcohol content (BAC), means that you can be arrested for "OUIL." OUIL stands for "operating a motor vehicle under the influence of intoxicating liquor."

Even if you weigh 200 pounds, three beers are enough to raise the blood alcohol level to qualify as impaired and unable to drive under the motor vehicle laws of many states. After drinking a six-pack in an hour, you would be considered legally drunk, according to the U.S. Department of Transportation, and would be seven times more likely to have an accident as someone who had not been drinking.

When you accept a driver's license, you are giving your consent to be tested for alcohol in your blood. If you refuse to take an alcohol test, your license may be suspended and points added to your driving record. If you are arrested for OUIL in some states, your driver's license can even be taken by the arresting officer and cut up on the spot. If you are convicted of OUIL, your license can be suspended for several months. You may also be fined and sentenced to jail and/or community service. When your suspension is over, you may have to pay to get your license back, if you can get it back at all.

Contract For Life

Kids who belong to Students Against Driving Drunk (SADD) believe there is no such thing as responsible use. Alcohol (if you are underage) and drug use are illegal. Period. To help keep you safe and alive, they urge you and your parents or guardian to sign the contract for life that appears on page 117.

Find Another Way Home

If you're out partying with someone who has been drinking or using drugs, it's up to you to find another way home. When the person insists they can drive, don't be fooled.

- Drive the person home.
- Ask someone else who's sober to drive you and the other person home.
- Call a taxi.
- Insist the person take a bus or the subway if it's available.
- Take away the person's key, if you have to.
- Call a parent or another adult to help.

How To Help A Friend Who Has Had Too Much

We were having a blast. Everyone was really drunk. A group of us pinned Kyle down, opened his mouth and just started pouring. He crashed. We thought it was funny until we realized he wasn't getting up.

BRAD, 17

Alcohol poisoning occurs when a lot of alcohol is consumed in a short span of time. Ten drinks can cause serious problems for most people. Fourteen drinks can kill them. You'll know someone is in danger when:

- he won't wake up and doesn't respond when talked to, shouted at, pinched or shaken

CONTRACT FOR LIFE

A FOUNDATION FOR TRUST & CARING

By agreeing to this contract, we recognize that SADD encourages all young people to adopt a **substance-free** life style. We view this contract as a means of opening the lines of communication about drinking, drug use and traffic safety to ensure the safety of all parties concerned. We understand that this contract does not serve as permission to drink, but rather, a promise to be safe.

Young Adult

I acknowledge that the legal drinking age is 21 and have discussed with you and realize both the legal and physical risks of substance use, as well as driving under the influence. I agree to contact you if I ever find myself in a position where anyone's substance use impairs the possibility of my arriving home safely. I further pledge to maintain safe driving practices at all times, including wearing my safety belt every trip and encouraging others to do the same.

Signature_____

Parent or Guardian

Upon discussing this contract with you, I agree to arrange for your safe transportation home, regardless of time or circumstances. I further vow to remain calm when dealing with your situation and discuss it with you at a time when we are *both* able to converse calmly about the matter.

I agree to seek safe, sober transportation home if I am ever in a situation where I have had too much to drink or a friend who is driving me has had too much to drink. Recognizing that safety belt usage is a vital defense against death and injury on the highway, I promise to wear my safety belt at all times and encourage others to do the same.

Signature_____

Date_____

Distributed by S.A.D.D. "Students Against Driving Drunk"

- his skin feels clammy and is a purplish color
- he is having trouble breathing
- he has a rapid or irregular heart beat

If you think a friend has overdosed on alcohol:
- don't leave them alone
- call 911 or a doctor as fast as you can
- lay the person on his or her side or sit them up with their head bowed, so they won't choke on their own vomit. (Alcohol is a poison, and one of the ways your body tries to get rid of it is by vomiting. Unfortunately, if a person vomits but is so drunk they can't cough and clear their airway, they can suffocate to death.)
- clear the mouth and breathing airway if the person has vomited
- provide first aid until help arrives

Marijuana: Point-blank

FACT: Marijuana is an illegal drug and can be psychologically addicting. Known as pot, dope, weed, grass, Mary Jane, ganja and reefer on the street, marijuana is a "gateway" drug. Part-time users often become all-the-time users or begin abusing "harder" drugs such as cocaine and LSD.

FACT: Marijuana contains more cancer causing agents than tobacco smoke and can damage the lungs because the smoke is inhaled and held in the lungs. One "joint" (marijuana cigarette) affects your lungs the same as 25 cigarettes.

FACT: Marijuana use may affect short-term memory and the ability to learn. It can screw up your sense of time and make it difficult for you to do things that require concentration and coordination.

FACT: Marijuana can make you feel anxious and paranoid, as if someone is watching you or out to get you.

FACT: In guys, marijuana can lower the level of testosterone—a hormone that controls hair and muscle growth and penis development. In girls, marijuana can increase the testosterone level which leads to more hair on the face and body and acne.

FACT: Using marijuana or hashish (a stronger form of the same drug) makes the heart beat faster, causes bloodshot eyes and a dry mouth and throat, and increases the appetite.

FACT: While you worry about the bad effects of the drug, you can also worry about the diseases, like hepatitis, that can be passed by sharing a joint or pipe.

The Effects Of Marijuana And Driving

People who use marijuana think they "can drive just fine, thank you." They can't. Marijuana affects a driver's ability in many of the same ways as alcohol, and the effects of the drug last for several hours after the feeling of being "high" passes. For example, some studies show that marijuana upsets:

- Muscle coordination. A driver who is "high" can have trouble controlling a vehicle quickly and correctly when necessary.

- Vision. Seeing double vision can be a problem with the glare of oncoming headlights.

- Tracking ability. The drug really affects your ability to track, or follow, a moving object with your eyes.

Smoking: Point-blank

FACT: Every day some 3,000 kids start smoking, and every day 1,000 smokers die.

FACT: Smoking kills more people than AIDS, car accidents, alcohol, murders, illegal drugs, suicides and fires *combined.*

FACT: Every cigarette steals seven minutes from a smoker's life. Every year, cigarettes steal a total of five million years from smokers' lives.

FACT: In some states it is illegal for anyone under 18 to have or use tobacco products, including cigarettes.

FACT: About half of all high school seniors who smoke cigarettes say they want to quit. Seven out of 10 young smokers say they wish they'd never started.

FACT: More teenagers prefer to date a nonsmoker than a smoker.

FACT: Nicotine, which is addictive, affects the brain and the central nervous system. It speeds up the heart beat, increases blood pressure and restricts the flow of blood to arms and legs.

FACT: Women who smoke and take birth control pills are at a greater risk for heart attack and stroke and may increase their chances of getting cancer of the cervix.

FACT: Cigarette smoke contains some 4,000 chemicals, some of which are known to cause cancer. Smoking is a major cause of cancers of the lung, mouth, larynx (voice box), esophagus (swallowing tube), stomach, bladder, kidney and cervix.

FACT: Inhaling secondhand smoke plays a part in asthma, allergies, cancer and other lung diseases.

FACT: Many of these diseases can be fatal (the chance of someone surviving lung cancer, even with treatment, is very low). Many of these diseases can also be prevented by quitting. Quitters may feel worse before they feel better. At first, they may feel tense and light-headed and have a cough and headaches. But in just hours, days and weeks, the body can begin to reverse the bad effects of smoking. After several years, the ex-smoker's risk of lung cancer or heart disease is about the same as someone's who never smoked at all.

Smokeless Tobacco: Point-blank

FACT: Smokeless tobacco, also known as snuff, a quid, a chew or a plug, is not safer than smoking cigarettes. The nicotine just comes in a different package. All tobacco causes cancer. It could happen sooner with smokeless tobacco—especially in the mouth, tongue, cheek, nose and gums.

FACT: Even before cancer develops from chewing, gums and lips can crack and bleed, and white patches and sores can develop inside the mouth. Tobacco also damages gums, stains the teeth and the smell of your breath could stop a train. ("Kiss me, nothing makes me sick.")

FACT: Chewing gives a "buzz" by speeding up the heart and raising blood pressure. After using snuff for only a short time, another dip will be needed every 20 to 30 minutes to keep the high going. Without another hit, a person may begin to feel dizzy, shaky and cranky.

Inhalants: Point-blank

FACT: Inhalants come in many forms: plastic cement, fingernail polish remover, lighter fluid, hair spray, cleaning products. Misuse of these products is illegal and can be deadly.

FACT: The effects of inhalants—which are sniffed and breathed in from bottles, cloths soaked in the inhalant or vapor-filled bags and balloons—can last for a few minutes up to an hour.

FACT: A person can get used to inhalants so that more of the drugs are needed to reach the same high. Hallucinations, chills, stomach cramps, headaches and the shakes are common withdrawal symptoms.

FACT: Though it may seem like just a harmless kick, inhalants decrease oxygen to the brain. If used for a long time, the user can feel sick to their stomach, vomit and have headaches (and this is the best you can expect—it gets much worse). Vapors can attack your liver, lungs and kidneys and damage your central nervous system.

FACT: Inhalants can stop your breathing. When a bag or balloon is used, a person can suffocate. Inhalants can also cause sudden death by stopping the heart from beating. A single hit could be your first—and your last.

FACT: If you're inhaling, STOP NOW! Some of these problems may be able to be reversed if you STOP NOW!

Cocaine/Crack: Point-blank

FACT: Even one hit of crack can kill. Even first-time users of cocaine can have seizures and heart attacks.

FACT: Crack is very habit-forming, even more so than heroin or barbiturates. Repeated use can lead to addiction within just a few days. Long-term use can result in violent behavior and mental problems like schizophrenia, where a person loses touch with reality.

FACT: Cocaine can be snorted through the nose, smoked (freebasing), or injected—and in each case is quickly absorbed into the brain and bloodstream.

FACT: When you inject cocaine, you may also be injecting hepatitis and the AIDS virus into your body.

FACT: Crack (rock) is cocaine that comes in the form of tiny chunks. It can be made with other chemicals which are also harmful and deadly.

FACT: A person on cocaine may at first feel energized and powerful but can quickly "crash" and become depressed and edgy.

FACT: Cocaine, in any form, including crack, excites the brain and central nervous system which may cause brain seizures, heart attack, respiratory (breathing) failure or stroke. The drug can also affect a person's ability to perform during sex.

FACT: Many users talk about "coke bugs" or the feeling that bugs are crawling all over their body.

FACT: Users spend a lot of money to support their illegal habit only to increase their risk of drowning, car accidents, falls, burns and suicide while on the drug.

Speed: Point-blank

FACT: Speed (amphetamine) does exactly what the name suggests. Users say the illegal substance makes them feel alert, happy and like they could go on forever. But they don't. Heavy use of speed can kill.

FACT: Speed, in the form of methamphetamine, diet pills and caffeine cuts the appetite, speeds up the heart rate, distorts thinking and can keep the user up for hours. Nervousness, confusion, aggressiveness, wild mood swings, hallucinations, paranoia, loss of coordination, eating disorders, the shakes, convulsions and brain damage can also occur on speed.

FACT: Speed is habit-forming. After awhile, a person needs more of the drug to get the same high or to avoid a bad "crash."

FACT: Withdrawal from speed can cause fatigue, stomach cramps and depression. Confusion and memory loss can continue for up to a year.

Hallucinogens/LSD/PCP/Ecstasy: Point-blank

FACT: Hallucinogens (or psychedelics) like PCP, LSD and Ecstasy twist reality. What you see, feel and do are not linked to what's real. Users lose control of their body and mind and often harm themselves or are violent toward others.

FACT: What will happen with each use is anybody's guess. The "trip" depends on the user's personality, the amount taken and whether he or she takes it at a party or alone. A "bad trip" can last for 12 hours. A user's

124 GET IT? GOT IT. GOOD!

body heats up, the heart rate jumps, and the person begins to sweat. Depression, panic, mood swings and scary hallucinations can also happen.

FACT: All of these illegal drugs are habit-forming. A user may need more and more of the drug to reach the same high. More of a bad thing can lead to a "bad trip," convulsions, coma, heart and lung failure, burns, falls, drowning and death.

LSD: Point-blank

FACT: You can't smell, see or taste LSD, or acid. Know what you're getting into when someone offers you a tablet or capsule or thin squares of jello (window panes) or small squares of paper (blotter acid).

FACT: LSD makes a user "break from reality" and feel anxious and depressed. Illusions and hallucinations are common with LSD. A person may think they can "see" music or "hear" colors.

Ecstasy: Point-blank

FACT: On ecstasy a user may feel on top of the world. Unfortunately, their brain isn't so lucky.

FACT: Ecstasy is used at "rave" parties (underground dance parties at which no alcohol is served but ecstasy is used) and has been called the "dance making" drug. Users have been known to move on a hot, crowded dance floor to the point of heatstroke, collapse, convulsions, coma, heart failure and death.

FACT: After even short-term use, the side effects of ecstasy include: sleeplessness, numbness, loss of appetite, jaw clenching and teeth grinding, headaches, nausea and depression. Users also suffer from hangovers the next day. They feel spent and can't do even simple tasks.

FACT: Ecstasy and LSD are sometimes used together (known as X-n-L) with the same dangerous results.

PCP: Point-blank

FACT: PCP, or angel dust, can create a feeling of well-being and numbness. Users can be excited and aggressive, or depressed, withdrawn and paranoid.

FACT: Confusion, memory loss, weight loss, an inability to think and learn, violent behavior and paranoia are also effects of PCP.

FACT: PCP comes in the form of "dust," pills, liquid and can be mixed with marijuana for smoking. The drug is habit-forming. Withdrawal makes a user have headaches, an increased need for sleep and a craving for more of the drug.

CAT: Point-blank

FACT: CAT, or methcathinone, is an illegal drug which is like cocaine but thought to be more powerful. On the street, it's referred to as Star, Wonder and Crank.

FACT: When someone injects, inhales or sprinkles CAT on marijuana and smokes it, they are invading their body with poison including ephedrine (a stimulant which revs up your system), battery acid, lye, paint thinner, epsom salts, acetone and muriatic acid.

FACT: Early CAT users say it makes them feel happy, full of energy and powerful. The bad part happens when these first highs dissolve into paranoia, depression, frightening hallucinations and violent behavior. CAT is also known to be habit-forming.

Heroin: Point-blank

FACT: Heroin, also known as junk, smack and horse, comes in a powder form that ranges in color from white to dark brown. Heroin can be injected ("mainlining"), snorted or smoked.

FACT: A feeling of well-being is the first effect of this illegal substance, followed by slowed heart rate, breathing and brain activity, nausea, drowsiness and a craving for more of the drug.

FACT: AIDS, blood poisoning and hepatitis can result from sharing needles to shoot heroin. Convulsions, coma and death from overdose are also common.

FACT: Withdrawal symptoms include chills, sweating, tremors, irritability and sleeplessness. These problems can last as long as 7-10 days.

Steroids: Point-blank

FACT: Anabolic steroids, taken with a program of muscle-building exercise and diet, may increase body weight and strength. But winning isn't worth it. If you use steroids, you're exposing yourself to more than 70 possible side effects ranging from liver cancer to acne, and some of these problems last forever.

FACT: In males, steroids can cause testicles to shrivel up. Guys may become impotent which means they can't keep an erection during sex and may also be unable to father children.

FACT: Females may become more masculine. Smaller breasts and an inability to conceive and have kids is also possible.

FACT: In both sexes, aggressive or violent behavior, depression, swelling of the feet and lower legs, darkening of the skin and constant bad breath can also occur. While some of these side effects appear quickly, others, such as heart attacks, cancer and strokes, may not show up for years.

Prescription Drugs: Point-blank

FACT: Medicines don't have the same effect on everybody and should never be taken by someone other than for whom they were prescribed.

FACT: Some medicines don't mix well with certain foods,

other medicines and alcohol. Ask your doctor or pharmacist before mixing.

FACT: Finish all of your medicine as ordered. Otherwise, you might get rid of the symptoms but not the entire problem. If at any time a medicine makes you feel bad or weird, gives you headaches, stomachaches, rashes or dizziness, tell your doctor right away.

FACT: Abusing any drug—including prescription ones—can lead to serious illness and death. Just because your doctor prescribed it for you doesn't mean the drug isn't dangerous if used the wrong way.

Do You Have A Drug Or Alcohol Problem?

If you or someone you know can answer "yes" to two or more of the following questions, it may be a sign that a drug and/or alcohol problem exists, and it's time to get help.

1. Are you drinking or using drugs to "quit hurting" or to hurt your mom and dad?
2. Does your drinking or using other drugs make it hard to get along with your friends?
3. Have you taken drinks or other drugs because you are shy and find it makes it easier to talk to people and have more fun at parties?
4. Are you unhappy or guilty about your drinking or drug use?
5. Does drinking or drugging make it tough for you to do well at school, or your job, in team sports or other activities?
6. Are you spending more time alone because of your drugs or drinking?
7. Are your friendships changing because of your drugs?
8. Do you have unexplained depression or anxiety or problems sleeping?
9. Has anybody, either jokingly or in seriousness, talked to you about your use?

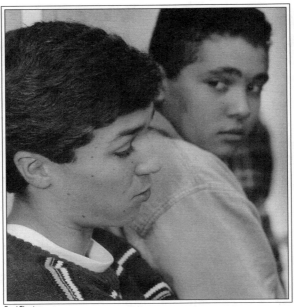

Brad Fleming

10. Do you need a drink or other drugs to have fun or feel comfortable on a date?

11. Are you hiding liquor, joints or drugs and lying about their use?

12. Do you need a drug or drink to quit shaking, to quiet down or for your nerves?

13. Do you need alcohol or other drugs to start your day?

14. Does your mom, dad, brother, sister or anyone in your close family have a problem with alcohol or drugs?

15. Have you ever had a loss of memory after drinking or taking drugs and have you ever done or said things you cannot remember?

16. Do you think about getting drunk or high all the time?

17. Do you steal so you can support your habit?

18. Have you lost control over how much you use?
19. Do you experience any signs of withdrawal when not drinking such as headaches, nausea, vomiting or "the shakes?"

AUTHOR UNKNOWN

When Substance Abuse Touches You

If a friend, relative or parent shows any of these signs, don't cover up and make excuses for the person, and don't blame yourself. Substance abuse is an addiction, and an addiction is a disease, like cancer. You cannot cause, control or cure a parent's drinking or drug problem. Neither can the millions of other Americans who grow up in homes with substance abusers.

Addicted parents are sick, not bad. They may deny they have a problem. They may say things they don't mean or forget things they have said or done. Yet, they can and do get well, with special help and your understanding and support.

You deserve help, whether or not your parent gets it. Protect yourself by not driving with a parent who is drunk. Stay out of the way if the person becomes abusive or violent, and keep phone numbers on hand of people to call in case of an emergency.

If your parents are drinking and taking drugs, learn from their mistake—don't use it as an excuse to start using yourself.

Whether the problem is with family or friends, don't try to handle things alone. Talk to someone you trust. It's not tattling, it's saving a life.

You Can Pursue Happiness. . .Elsewhere

You don't need drugs to have fun. I want to remember my weekends. I want to remember my high school years, rather than spend them in a bottle.

BECKY, 19

It's easy to convince yourself nothing bad is going to happen if you "partake." To say "sure" when your friends ask you to have a drink or smoke some pot. Besides, you want to find out what it's all about. You want to fit in and be liked.

Wanting to feel good and have friends is not a crime, but you can do it without hurting yourself. If you don't want to get high and your friends do, here are some ways to say "NO":

- tell them "thanks, but no thanks"

- have the courage to walk away

- come up with something else for everybody to do

- be a broken record—each time you're asked to join in, say "No"—your "so-called friends" will get tired of hearing it

- avoid the situation altogether

- give a reason or excuse (like you're the designated driver)

When The Pressure Is On

Peer pressure only exists if you let it exist. Some kids feel the only way to be cool is by doing what the others are doing. If I get pressured into something I don't want to do, I try to remove myself from the situation as soon as possible. This may mean that I'm not so cool, but if I'm happy with what I've done, that's all that matters.

TIFFANY, 17

- Remember, friends don't ask friends to do things that hurt them.

- Ask yourself why—maybe they're pushing you because they want your okay for something they know is wrong—sort of a twist on "misery loves company."

- Talk to someone you trust.

- Get some exercise.

Natural Highs

Swimming the last lap. Christmas carols. A long distance call from a friend. Good grades. Water-skiing. A hug. Your team winning. Listening to a child giggle. Watching a sunset. Your heartbeat when you see someone you like. Watching a cat take a bath in a patch of sun. Intercepting a pass. Eating pizza. A long, hot shower. A spider web with dew on it in the early morning sun. A great book. Reading under an electric blanket on a rainy day. Your first solo bike ride. Intimacy. A good talk with a friend. A great idea. Snow skiing. A kitten. Enthusiastic people. Climbing trees. Watching the moon. Plunging your hot body into a cool pool. Running in the fall. Relaxing to Saturday morning cartoons. Making somebody laugh. Surfing. Walking on the beach. Decorating a Christmas tree. Playing the piano. Sailing. Fixing something that's been broken. A job well done. Creativity. Football. Slumber parties. Liking your parents. The quiet after a snowfall. Riding down the street in a sports car switching gears. Friends. Singing. Really observing things. A letter from a friend. Color. Frisbee. Being appreciated. Losing weight. Being noticed by somebody you've been noticing. A warm smile from a stranger. Success stories. Dancing. Finishing a term paper. The first week of school. The last week of school. The day the yearbook comes out. Laughter. Recognizing the truth in something you read. Hearing somebody say, "I love you." Holding hands. Clean hair. Stopping smoking. The first spring flower. Loving yourself.

Adapted from "Bridging the Gap." Reprinted in: "The Parent Line" 1987 Vol. IV #3 Prevention Services, Ionia, MI

- Reward yourself by doing something special—shop, go to a movie, shoot hoops, rollerblade.

- Think of something you like—the last day of school and the first day of summer.

- Get with a different group of friends—there are other people out there just like you—with your interests, your feelings, your attitudes—find them and have fun.

- Plan a "chemical-free" party of your own, have things to do that don't include alcohol, and don't allow "gate-crashers."

- Bring your own soft drinks to parties (Sprite looks a lot like a gin and tonic...who's to know, and why should you care?!).

- Accept a beer, go to the bathroom, pour it out, fill the can with water and go party.

- Make a pact with a friend not to drink at the party and help each other keep the promise.

- Get high on the party and see how crazy you can get without alcohol and drugs.

- Remember...you can always get help from a responsible adult.

- For more information and program materials for use in your high school, write or call MADD (Mothers Against Drunk Driving) or SADD (Students Against Driving Drunk).

  MADD
  511 E. John Carpenter Freeway, Suite 700
  Irving, Texas 75062
  1-800-GET-MADD

  SADD
  P.O. Box 800
  Marlboro, Massachusetts 01752
  (508) 481-3568

Where You Can Find Help

You have a lot to lose. Your self-respect, your dignity, your mom and dad, your family's trust. True friends. A good education. A chance to find the love of your life. Your freedom. A future. Your life. Alcohol and drugs can take this all away from you.

Help is within your reach. There are people who care about you. People who have dedicated their lives to helping others who are addicted to alcohol and drugs. Some of them are ex-addicts, like Melba, who can give first-hand details about that side of life. There are also your parents, relatives, counselors and teachers at school, ministers, priests or rabbis and family friends.

Other great people can be found in community mental health centers, hospitals, halfway houses, family service agencies, private physicians' and therapists' offices, specialized alcohol treatment clinics, and crisis and recovery centers. Self-help support groups like AA (Alcoholics Anonymous), NA (Narcotics Anonymous), Alateen and Narateen also offer friendship, support and help in coping with your own addiction, a friend's or a family member's.

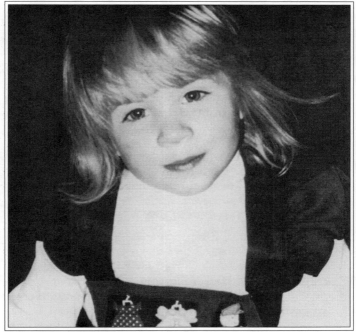

AD Council/U.S. Dept. of Transportation

8

Andy Pandy

*The car spun and spun. It was as if everything was
in slow motion. I thought I would die, but I didn't.
No, instead, Mike S. spared my life. He tried to
pass on the left because passing on the right would
have ruined the boat. You and your mommy were
on the right. So, now I am the historian of the
collision that took your life.*

Your mommy and I went to order a cake for your big sister. Amy's 14th birthday was the next day. You wanted to go, too, so of course, your mommy let you. You were so easy to look at. So easy to love.

We were gone only 20 minutes or so. Only downtown to the bakery. We were stopped, waiting to make a left turn into your driveway. We were "home." I unfastened my seat belt, and I started to turn towards you so I could say, "we're home" in that singsong voice that adults always use with small children. Because of your injuries, I now know that you were already looking "home." The coroner said your head was turned that way. We're home, Andy Pandy. We're home.

Your mommy was unconscious. She had been hit so hard that she was having a brain seizure. God, you were so still. Your little head was resting on your chest. Part of me said, "she's asleep," and part of me said, "she's dead." But I didn't really say anything. I was too busy screaming.

Your daddy was there. He ran down the driveway and across the street. He broke out the window to the back seat and put his mouth over yours. He puffed little breaths of life into your lungs until the paramedics and fire department came. Between those puffs, I heard him say over and over, "Oh God, my baby, my baby! Oh God, my baby!"

I lay in emergency next to your mommy, and I heard the doctor tell your daddy your head was cracked like an egg. But all the king's horses and all the king's men couldn't put Andy together again.

I waited in intensive care, and I saw the doctors tell your mommy you were dead. Brain dead. Your mommy cried and begged everyone, "Tell me it's not true! Oh why? Oh why? Tell me it's not true!"

Someone brought a paper for your mommy to sign, and they took your mommy into a room with your daddy. After a long time, they came out.

Your mommy cried and begged the nurses to let her lie down with you. And they did. They moved all the tubes and monitors, and they made a space for your mommy on the bed next to you. All the nurses cried.

Your mommy cried and cried and begged everyone, "Tell me it's not true! Oh why? Tell me it's not true!

I stood at the end of your bed, and I watched your mommy kiss every inch of you. And touch every inch of you. And inhale the smell of you. For eight hours.

The machines that made your lungs breathe glowed with a blue-green glow. The color of the car that hit us. Fueled by alcohol. Over three times the legal limit.

Sara and your daddy had to pull your mommy off your body. It was eight hours after you had been pronounced dead and three days since the crash.

Your mommy screamed and screamed and cried and cried and begged everyone, "Tell me it's not true! Oh, why? Tell me it's not true!"

A man without a heart took your heart from you. He broke your mommy's and daddy's heart for eternity.

It was as if Mike S. had stopped his car and beat you over the head with a beer can.

In a heartbeat, Mike S. took all of your chances away from you.

No kindergarten. No first grade. No more horse shows. No more scraped knees. No high school. No prom. No first love. No college. No marriage. No babies. No grandchildren.

Only a grave. And no heart.

We do not know what your heart might have been able to accomplish had you been allowed to keep it.

And in a heartbeat, Mike S. changed all of our lives forever.

Forever and ever, when I close my eyes, I will hear Jim Harris say over and over, "Oh God, my baby, my baby! Oh God, oh God, my baby!"

And forever and ever, when I close my eyes, I will hear Carol Harris cry over and over and beg everyone, "Tell me it's not true! Oh why? Oh why? Tell me it's not true!"

Thank you Mike S....forever and ever and ever.

A four-year-old child...you are in my heart forever, Andy. Forever and ever and ever...

In loving memory of Andrea Lee Harris.
Awaited with joy, welcomed with love May 20, 1987.
Taken from our lives August 26, 1991.

R. STEINBERG, A FRIEND OF ANDY'S MOMMY AND A PASSENGER IN THE CAR THAT DAY IN AUGUST 1991.

Drunk Driving Is No Accident

For perhaps the first time in the history of the United States, a drunk driver, Mike S., was charged, not with vehicular manslaughter, but second-degree murder. This guilty verdict is paving the way for a new attitude in this country: drunk driving deaths are no accident.

The seat belt Andy Harris was wearing couldn't save her life, but saved the lives of four people. One life saved for each year she lived. A five-year-old boy runs and plays with Andy's heart and lungs. One of her kidneys was donated to a one-year-old, the other to a fifty-four-year-old. A three-year-old is living a full life with Andy's liver.

Carol Harris continues to work tirelessly to stop drunk driving deaths through her local chapter of RID (Remove Intoxicated Drivers) and P.M.O.C. (Parents of Murdered Children and Other Survivors of Homicide Victims).

Vows Carol, "I'm not finished yet."

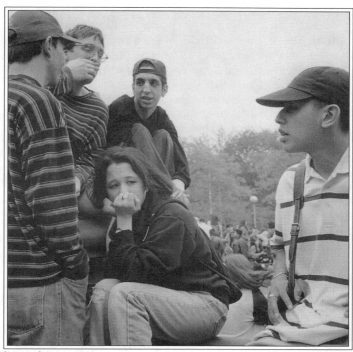
Christopher Smith, Impact Visuals

9

When The Heat Is On

In an average hour on an average day:
- 10 women are raped
- 240 women are beaten by their husbands or boy-friends
- 330 burglaries are committed
- 129 people are assaulted
- 3 people are murdered

Nearly two million violent crimes are reported every year in the United States. According to the Bureau of Justice Statistics, teenagers are the targets of crime more than any other group. In fact, they're not only the victims in most cases, but the criminals.

Why do these bad things have to happen?

There are a lot reasons. People's differences over race, religion and sex can provoke violence. A person without any self-esteem may attack others to prove his or her own power. Some people have mental problems that they can't control. Yet, none of these reasons are a good excuse for violence. There is no excuse.

Maybe you know violence firsthand. Is there someone you know who is abused at home, who carries a gun to school, or has been hurt by a violent person or gang? Are you that person?

Fight The Violence, Not The Person

When someone hurts or threatens you, you have two choices: fight the person or fight the violence. Using violence to stop violence is like fighting fire with fire. It's like the old saying goes: "what goes around, comes around."

To fight violence, the first thing you have to do is realize that it's wrong. No matter who is violent or where or why, it's wrong. At home, in the country or on the streets of a big city.

Stop Accepting Violence

It's a funny thing about life; if you refuse to accept anything but the best, you very often get it.
SOMERSET MAUGHAN

You don't have to accept violence! Giving in and giving up just puts more power back into the hands of people who should never have it.

• So, tune out and turn off. Watching violence on

TV, listening to it on a CD and pretending to do it day after day on video games make it seem just a normal part of everyday life. No way!

People bleed in real life. They don't get up after being shot or beaten to death. They lose their chance to fall in love, get married, have children, and be happy, forever. And forever is much longer than the time it takes for the show to be over.

- Value yourself and others as individuals, not just a group of people of a certain race, religion or sex.

- Take a look at people who have changed the world for the better, and follow their lead. These people didn't get where they wanted to go by using violence. They used a great idea, an open mind, a kind heart and a belief in basic human values like compassion, equality, honesty and hard work.

- Maybe you can't control what other people do, but you can control who your friends are. Stay away from people, places and situations you think or know are trouble.

- Be strong enough to tell a friend, "Hey, I'm not hanging with you until you ditch the tool (weapon), because I know where that's going." This kind of attitude may cost you a few friends. It may make you uncool, but we're talking survival here. You know where violence leads—to the hospital, to prison or into the ground. If you have any hopes and dreams in your life, don't accept it.

- Find out the real truth about gangs. Kids join them because they can't seem to find love, security, acceptance and a sense of family at home, at school or in their hometown or neighborhood. Sadly, these kids end up tied to a life of violence and crime.

If you're in a gang, death is one way out. So is being sent to prison. Some members are "jumped out," which means they are badly beaten by other gang members. If they're still alive when it's all over,

they've earned their freedom. Many gangs respect
achievement, so going with a "steady" girlfriend or
boyfriend, getting a job, going to school or excel-
ling in sports may also provide another way out.

- Start a "gang" of your own or join a group of other
  kids and adults who feel the same way you do about
  violence.

- Learn how to control your own anger and solve
  problems peacefully.

When The Heat Is On

At some, or many, points in your life, you're gong to butt
heads with somebody else. Whether it's because you're
mad, scared, frustrated, hurt or disappointed, one thing's
for sure...you're ready to blow!

The first step to controlling your anger is no step at
all. In fact, STOP...whatever you're doing and whatever
you're thinking.

- Count to 10. Backwards.

- Think about the most important person in your life
  at this exact moment. (Yeah, you.) Sort out all
  your feelings. Ask yourself: "Why am I angry? What
  happened that made me feel this way? What did
  the person do? What did I do? How important is
  this issue anyway? Do I really want to waste my
  time and energy on being angry?"

- You have to control your anger before you can control the situation. If you can't get control, get away.
  Take a time out. Find the calm before the storm.

- Realize it's okay to be angry, but it's not okay to
  throw a punch. Set the record straight firmly without hurting someone else or getting hurt yourself.

- Think about the options and consequences of your
  actions. You could hit somebody, but it's only going to get you more of the same and could ruin any
  chances at a good, long relationship with the other

person. If you like your face the way it is, check your anger at the door. There are better ways to solve problems that won't lay you out or land you in jail.

The trick is to find ways of letting off steam without causing harm. Have a shaving cream or water balloon fight to settle differences with a friend. Challenge the person to a game of skill or a race. Flip a coin to decide who is right. Find something funny about the whole situation and laugh it off. Put the person's picture in your shoes and walk around on their face for a while.

Now That You've Cooled Off

How do you best solve the problem?

- Make sure you've counted to 10 enough times, and then speak up and help the other person do the same. Silence has never solved a problem.

- Hear the person out. Listen carefully. Where are they coming from? What are their needs? Maybe you don't know the whole story or the reason behind what happened. You can't solve the problem until you understand the person. As Albert Einstein said: "Peace cannot be kept by force. It can only be achieved by understanding."

- Be assertive, not aggressive. Stand up for your ideals, but don't shove them down somebody else's throat. Never attack the person by pointing fingers, name-calling or placing blame. Begin every sentence with "I." "I feel this way" or "I would like the solution to be..." rather than "you." "You are nothing but a liar," or "You better change your stupid ways."

- Don't bring up past problems which don't have any connection to the situation at hand. You'll just be adding fuel to the fire. Deal with one issue at a time.

- Make sure the way you stand, hold yourself and

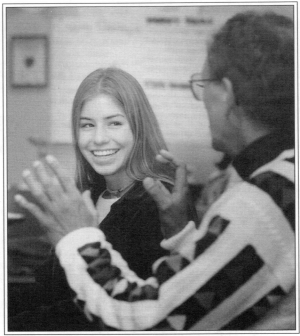

Brad Fleming

speak lets the other person know you're open-minded and willing to work toward a compromise.

- Be willing to admit and be responsible for something you may have done wrong.

- Respond with your head, not your fists. Your brain is specially designed to think, analyze and solve problems. Brainstorm together. Find out the facts and then find a common solution in which everybody wins.

Resolving conflict is not always going to work. It involves other people, and everyone must want to play by the rules. If it looks hopeless, be smart enough to keep your cool. If the other person doesn't want to go along, accept that and carry on. Never lose sight of your main goal: peace.

The Other Option Is Not Pretty

The courts are gettin' tougher on us. The way it is now, kids are gonna wish they were being tried as kids. At least when you're young, they try to help you get your head on straight. When you go to prison as an adult, you've hit a dead end.

Ty, 16, #529677

The magic age in a court of law is about 17 or 18 years old. That's the age when you can be tried as an adult. Even younger kids, like Ty, can be tried as adults for crimes like murder, rape and armed robbery.

Every state has different laws, but the "juvenile justice system" usually has three levels: probation, detention, prison. And each one is a kid's own worst nightmare.

Probation

If you're under probation, you may be allowed to stay at home, but there'll be some heavy limits on where you go, who you see and what you do. You'll feel like your parents and probation officer are breathing down your neck.

Probation may involve random testing if drugs are involved. You may also have to:

- complete an educational program
- pay for damages or stolen items
- counsel face-to-face with the victim
- perform community service work
- attend rehabilitation programs on topics like drug abuse, controlling anger and resolving conflict.

Detention

If you're sentenced to detention, you may be taken from your home overnight or for a few days to live in another home that gives you zip, zero, nada, nothing privileges. If you are taken from you're home to a foster home, you can expect to be there for a longer time. If you are sentenced to live in a youth residential facility, you will not only be moved out of your home for several months, but may also be taken out of your community or neighborhood.

Mom And Dad Aren't Going To Be Happy

Your mistake may very well cost your parents, too. Not only will they be sad, angry and disappointed, but they may also have to pay for your actions. Your parents can be hit up for hundreds or thousands of dollars to cover property damage, lawyer and court fees, probation charges, foster or residential care and jail time. They may have to attend parenting classes, be restricted from leaving their own home or town or even go to jail themselves.

What Happens To You Depends Upon You

Your attitude may be the most important thing when it comes to deciding your fate. If you can prove there is little chance you'll break the law again, that you're willing to go to counseling and get help from others, and that you're not a risk to the community, you'll fare much better in the juvenile justice system.

Remember you can put yourself there, you can keep yourself out.

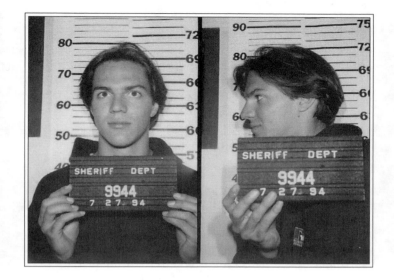

10

Advice From Inside

Larry and John started out as good kids. They were smart, happy and had real hopes for the future. Today, they are known as prisoners #145972 and #157475. They have some advice for you.

Lawrence Swearington

I'm not sure why I committed my first offense. I think I was about 7 or 8 years old. I stole candy bars from the store. I wasn't caught, so I wasn't punished.

Since then I have committed shoplifting,

burglary, peeping into neighbor's windows and sexual assault (rape).

I guess there are a lot of reasons I turned to crime. The first was because I wanted things I couldn't afford. I wasn't poor. I just didn't want to work for what I wanted. To me, it was easier to take it than to work for it.

When I was young, I also suffered from low self-esteem. My childhood wasn't any better or worse than the next person's. What was different was the way I looked at my life. Because of low self-esteem I let problems become bigger than they should have been. I kept a lot of feelings in. These same feelings would come out of me in anger and in a need to control some part of my life. I raped a woman out of anger at the way I felt I was treated by society. I also felt a need to make up for a feeling of having no control over my life.

My latest sentencing was for breaking and entering a home and raping the woman who lived there. Two days after committing this offense, on July 21, 1975, I was in prison.

The first thing I felt was fear of the unknown. I was sent to Jackson Prison (State Prison of Southern Michigan.) I didn't know what to expect living behind the walls of "The World's Largest Walled Prison."

There are many reasons to be afraid of living in prison. Make no mistake about it. There's a lot of violence in here. Sometimes it happens so fast, you don't even know why. Knowing that it does happen and you could get hurt bad is a thought that stays with you all the time. Living under all of that pressure is stressful. Once you've been in prison, the experience stays with you for the rest of your life.

Without question, the worst thing about living in prison is the loneliness that settles in shortly after arriving and doesn't leave until you're released.

On the outside, you have family, loved ones and friends who want to help you not harm you. Once you're separated from them, you're surrounded by hundreds of strangers who could care less about you. Most inmates want and will take whatever they can from whomever they can.

Another terrible thing about prison life is that time passes on without you. Since I have been in prison, my wife has divorced me, and my daughter has grown from an eight-year-old child to a twenty-seven-year-old woman. My father died. And then my mother died twelve years later. There is so much I wanted to tell them before they died. Now, I will never have the chance.

Relationships don't last long while in prison. A girlfriend or boyfriend on the outside will only wait so long before they'll want a "real" relationship with someone who can hold them and talk to them when they need it. You can't do that from prison. Prison is a lonely life.

My friends and family also suffer because I'm in prison. They may not talk about how hard it's been for them, but they suffer because you're not there for them. Slowly you grow apart, because they're on the outside, and you're on the inside. Your family is embarrassed every time someone asks about you. No one wants people to know that their son, daughter, cousin, aunt or uncle is in prison. Can you imagine having to tell your friends that your dad or mom is in prison?

Every day I am in prison, my family is in prison with me. Thankfully, my parents are spared any further shame because they are dead. The rest of the family lives on in shame. I could have avoided this trap by understanding how my actions affect other people – the victim and her family, and my family. I don't want to hurt anyone again.

If given the opportunity to turn back the clock and live time all over again, I would not commit any crimes. But that could only happen if I knew then what I know now. Now I have a good idea of the pain and suffering a victim and their family go through. I don't want to be the one responsible for creating another victim.

When my daughter was a teenager, I told her how life is in prison. I told her how a person's dignity is stripped from them. We are told what we can and can not do. Sometimes we're even told we can't go to the bathroom, because the officer doesn't want anyone walking around at a certain time.

Prison also steals a person's freedom and privacy. Do you think it's bad when your parents tell you that you have to stay in and can't go out? That happens everyday, every hour here.

Have your parents ever told you to do something that you didn't want to do? That happens all the time here, too. When a corrections officer tells you to do something, you have to do it whether you like it or not. If you don't do it-- you are in trouble. Getting in trouble here means that you may not be able to be released when you're supposed to be.

There is no guarantee a person who goes to prison will ever make it out. Prisoners kill prisoners. There are also prisoners who can't take it any longer and take their own lives. It's easy to think you would never take you own life. But it's another thing to live in prison day after day and put up with the madness. It just isn't worth it. Learn from my lesson, there is nothing fun about crime. It just doesn't pay.

The one thing I do have in my life is someone I can talk with about the things that are bothering me. I didn't find this "best friend" until I was in prison, and I found God. Having a person to talk with can help you get rid of the frustrations that will come about in your life. Without someone you can trust, anger can build until it is out of control. We all need someone—a dad, mom, brother, sister, aunt, uncle, teacher, minister or a good friend—that we can talk to.

LAWRENCE SWEARINGTON, PRISONER #145972, IS SERVING A SENTENCE FOR BREAKING AND ENTERING AND SEXUAL ASSAULT. HE HAS BEEN IN PRISON SINCE 1975 AND IS CURRENTLY HOUSED AT THE KINROSS CORRECTIONAL FACILITY.

John McKinnon

I can't remember the exact time I committed my first crime. As a juvenile, I got into a lot of mischief by doing things like stealing watermelons and breaking street lights. I began with these small crimes, but soon I was breaking into people's homes. I committed many crimes of breaking and entering (B&E). I finally made a mistake (as you always will), and I was caught.

My first B&E led to a 5-year prison sentence. I'm now 45 years old, with a total of 6 convictions for B&E, and I have been in prison for over 13 years.

I committed these crimes because I was trying to fit into the crowd. I gave in to pressure from my friends. It's something every kid has to deal with. I also used poor judgment. I committed crime to support my drug habit.

It is hard to explain what prison is like. Just as in the free world, life in prison is different for everyone. Every inmate deals with his sentence and the amount of time he has to serve in his own way. What you need to understand is that in prison there is a class structure just like in the free world. If a prisoner has to serve a natural life sentence, he will be exiled to a maximum security penitentiary where his every move will be closely guarded. In my case, I am in a minimum security facility. The killings, the stickings, the robberies and the gang rapes occur mostly in the higher security levels, though not always. There are prisoners at every level who are capable of trouble. If an inmate thinks he can get away with something, he will most likely try it.

Exercise (running, weight-lifting, walking) is a great way to deal with life here. There's so much "free" time we have to fill up, and yet we still need to feel like our lives are worth something. It would be easy for a prisoner to just sit around and eat and smoke. And that's what many of us do, waiting to die. Of course, in prison, a person doesn't have many choices. You can get trapped, so you no longer have the will to fulfill your goals in life.

Rehabilitation, which is supposed to make you a better person than the one who came in, isn't really offered in the adult prison system. Instead, it's up to the individual to try to work their way back into society. Basically, an inmate is responsible for his or her own rehabilitation.

I think the worst thing about being in prison is the total lack of privacy. If you have never experienced it, you could never understand. Both male and female officers observe you while you are in the shower and while you dress and undress. You're living in a place where you can't even shed a tear without everyone seeing it. I live with six other men in a space built for two. So, as you can see, the only way I'll gain any privacy is through parole.

Another tough thing about prison is the total separation from your family and friends. Being around people your whole life gives you fulfillment, and in prison that fulfillment is just torn away. Many prisoners have a hard time dealing with the fact that they're "out of sight, out of mind." We're left out of our family life and out of the real world. The longer the sentence, the more distant your family becomes.

In my eight years of prison life, I've had only two visits. One of these was to tell me that my sister had died. Being in prison has put a great deal of distance between my family and me, and I doubt I will ever be able to forgive them for abandoning me when I needed their support the most.

If I had it all to do over again, I would not make the same decisions that I made the first time. But you can't undo what's come before—not in prison and not in the free world.

The advice I want to give you is to learn the laws and follow them. If you start out as a child trying to push the system, you form a pattern that disregards the values that tell you right from wrong. When you develop a bad attitude toward the law, you start thinking the world revolves around you and the rules you make up. That's about the time you'll wake up in prison.

Don't "live for today"—plan for tomorrow. I can never get back my yesterdays, and I hope you haven't become so shallow that it takes a 45-year-old inmate's advice to keep you from becoming corrupt. I am a perfect example of the wrong way to live. Listen to what your Mom and Dad are telling you. They will lead you in the right direction.

JOHN LLOYD MCKINNON, PRISONER #157475, IS HOUSED AT THE MID-MICHIGAN CORRECTIONAL FACILITY AND IS SERVING A 10-15 YEAR SENTENCE AND A 9-30 YEAR SENTENCE FOR BREAKING AND ENTERING (B&E).

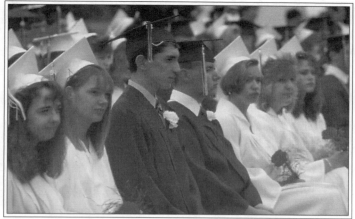

Jack Kurtz, Impact Visuals

11

All The Right Moves

The future always seems to arrive before you are ready to give up the present.

AUTHOR UNKNOWN

The Future Is Now

Why should I start planning my future now?

The future may seem like a long way off, but the decisions you make today can affect the rest of your life.

What kind of grades you get in high school will have an effect on what college you get into or the job you'll land right out of school. Your experience on the job or in college may help you begin a lifelong career. It will surely make a difference on how much money you can earn. College graduates, for example, can make up to twice as much on the job compared to those who don't attend or complete college. Your job may affect where and how well you live, who you meet and marry, the lives of your children, and on and on.

You must always strive for things ahead of you to make any progress in life. So, now is the time to ask yourself some questions and set some future goals:

- What do I want in life (success, respect, love, fun)?
- How can I achieve these things?
- Where do I want to be in 5 or 10 years?
- What's the best way to get where I want to go?
- What kind of skills and experience will I need?
- What can I do today, tomorrow and next week to help me reach my goals?

For example, if you think you want to be a doctor, here are some things you might want to do:

- believe in yourself
- work extra hard in chemistry, biology and health classes
- enter science fairs
- talk with a doctor and find out what it's all about
- get a job in a doctor's office
- volunteer at a hospital

Even staying on the right side of the law and keeping your body and mind healthy can affect your chances of being what you want to be.

I'm a high school junior this year and worried about what's out there for me after I graduate. Where do I start?

First of all, don't beat yourself over the head if you're not sure what you want to do the rest of your life. Most people don't have any idea either and end up changing their minds many times . . . so join the crowd.

Next, make a list of your interests and skills. Go back over every success you have had in your life including hobbies, grades and jobs, and write down the skills that helped you achieve these things.

Check to see if your school offers career interest surveys which can give you a list of careers and jobs that match your interests. Then talk with your high school guidance counselor about continuing education, college or career options available to you.

What if I choose to go to college?

College selection may be one of the most important decisions you and your parents will make. Take your time, you have a lot to think about.

Before you choose, decide what your goals are. What career interests do you have? How long do you want to be in school? Do you like classroom work, hands-on education or a little of both?

Make a list of what's important to you in terms of: location, size, courses, cost, athletics, social life and student activities.

If there is a college where you live, see if they offer dual enrollment programs. Dual enrollment means you can enroll in one or more of their college courses during the high school year. Sometimes you can earn both high school and college credit for the courses you complete. It's a good way to prepare yourself for full-time college. It's also a good way to test the field for career ideas.

How do I find out about different colleges?

No two colleges are exactly alike. A trip to your high school guidance counselor is a good place to begin for answers to your questions. You can also borrow or buy a college handbook from your public library or book store. These books can tell you all about American colleges and universities, admission requirements, testing information and financial aid. (Remember to look into both two and four-year colleges.) If you have access to a computer, there are also software programs that can give you this information.

Begin your college search as early as your junior year. You'll want to use that time to research colleges, visit campuses, take the required tests, fill in missed or required courses and sort out all of the options available to you. A junior year search also allows time to look into financial aid.

If you find some colleges you think would be right for you, call or visit the admissions office. Grab a college catalogue and newspaper. Talk to students who have been there. Go roam around campus. Tour the dorm rooms and even sit in on some classes. Check out the bulletin boards for an inside look at what goes on behind the scenes. While you're there you might also want to schedule an interview at the admissions office. Call ahead to make an appointment.

How does the college admissions process work?

After you send in your application, a record of your grades, high school activities and any other required information is sent directly from your high school to the college.

Colleges want students who can succeed, and they look at many things to predict how well you'll do:

- the reputation of your high school
- grades
- SAT, ACT and achievement test scores
- honors courses
- recommendations from teachers, coaches, employers, counselors
- one-on-one interviews
- school activities like band, peer counseling, debate club, creative arts
- community or church involvement
- special talents

- if any of your family attended the same college
- a personal essay describing yourself

A personal essay? What am I supposed to say?

Colleges are not only looking for good students, but for leaders and kids who have a desire to succeed as well. In a personal essay, you'll want to paint a picture of yourself that shows you are a good communicator, a leader, and a person with values like honesty, respect and hard work. Focus on the things that will set you apart from other college wanna-bes.

Depending upon what the application calls for, write about a major change in your life and how you handled it. Relate how you took a job and helped to improve the company overall. Talk about the future and how it will be a better place because you're in it. Don't lay it on too thick. College admission personnel have heard it all before. Just be honest about yourself and your accomplishments.

How many schools should I apply to?

There's no set number, but don't go hog wild and send in 100. That gets into some real money. (Application fees can run anywhere from $25.00 to $50.00 depending upon the school. Ask your guidance counselor about qualifying for local financial aid to cover these fees.) Some people say two or three is enough. Your guidance counselor will let you know how many is best for you.

If you have your heart set on a special place, apply— even if you think you can't get in. If you're not accepted at the college of your choice or can't get financial aid, the world as you know it isn't over. It's just delayed a bit. Try combining community college and work for a year. Then re-apply. Your success may show college admission officers you're ready for their program.

What are the SAT, ACT and achievement tests all about?

The Scholastic Aptitude Test (SAT) and the Achievement Test are part of the College Board's Admission Testing Program (ATP).

The SAT has a "verbal" section which measures reading comprehension (how much and how well you understand what you read) and vocabulary. A math section measures your skill with numbers and related concepts.

The SAT provides a way to rate you in comparison with other students from across the nation. SAT scores, plus a student's high school record, are used to predict a student's academic performance at the college level.

Achievement tests are designed to measure a student's ability in certain courses. A student can choose from fifteen one-hour tests on specific subject matters.

The American College Testing Program (ACT) is designed to test a student's general educational development and ability to handle college-level work in English, mathematics, reading and science reasoning. Students need to prove their knowledge and problem-solving and reasoning skills.

There is also the Preliminary Scholastic Aptitude Test (PSAT) which is a short version of the SAT. This test provides the experience of taking the SAT and is also used for qualification in the National Merit Scholarship.

Your guidance counselor can give you more information on testing dates, fees and financial aid to help cover costs.

How much emphasis is put on these test scores?

The College Entrance Examination Board believes a good school record is the single most important part of a student's application to college. However, these tests help the school determine the potential success of the student.

When do I take these tests?

These tests can be taken at the end of your junior year or in the senior year. Your guidance counselor can inform you of the specific test dates.

Is there any way to prepare for these tests?

Before you take these tests, you should know how they are organized, the kinds of questions that will be asked, the words and concepts used, and how they are timed and scored.

Many tests, such as the SAT and ACT, have booklets or computer programs which can help you prepare. Study the sample questions and make sure you understand the test directions. Then take the practice test, score it and review the questions you missed.

I want to go to college. But how can I pay for all of this?

Once again, your wizard of a high school guidance counselor can give you more information and the necessary forms to apply for financial aid.

Financial aid is based on merit, need or a combination of both. Merit-based financial aid is awarded to students who do very well in their studies, sports, leadership, music, art or dance. Need-based aid is awarded to students who wouldn't be able to continue their education past high school because of a lack of money.

How much money you get depends on the type of loan, whether it's based on academic success or financial need, and how much money the school has available for aid.

Financial Aid

There are many financial aid opportunities offered to students and parents of students who want to go to private, public, vocational and non-profit schools. These opportunities fall into the following categories: scholarships, loans, grants and work-study programs.

You don't have to pay back the money you get from scholarships and grants. These aids are usually awarded on the basis of academic achievement (how well you did in high school) and/or financial need.

Loans are monies that have to be repaid after leaving school. You probably will have to prove financial need before you can get a loan.

Work-study programs involve part-time work during the school year and full-time work during vacation periods. Again, proving that you need aid is sometimes necessary to get into these programs.

What do I need to apply for financial aid?

You must have a high school diploma or a General Education Development (GED) (see page 168) to receive financial aid.

All families must complete a Free Application for Federal Student Aid (FASFA). This application is used to figure your "expected family contribution (EOC)." A financial aid administrator will take the cost of your attendance and subtract the amount you and your family are expected to contribute toward that cost. If there's anything left over, you are proven to have financial need.

You can get an application from your guidance counselor's office or at any local community college or university financial aid office. Some schools may also require a Financial Aid Form. You must re-apply for financial aid every year.

Federal Aid Programs

The U.S. Department of Education offers the following financial aid programs.

- Federal Pell Grant Program. This grant is awarded on the basis of financial need to undergraduate students who have not earned a bachelor's or professional degree in fields like pharmacy or dentistry.

- Federal Supplemental Educational Opportunity Grant (FSEOG). This grant is awarded to undergraduate students who are most in need of financial aid and is often given to those who receive the Federal Pell Grant.

- Federal Work Study (FWS). The FWS is awarded to needy graduate and undergraduate students willing to work on or off campus to help pay for college. The program encourages community service and jobs related to the student's field of study.

Loans

- Federal Perkins Loan. This is a low interest loan for both undergraduate and graduate students who show strong financial need. This loan must be repaid. The amount you will owe depends upon the amount of the loan and the repayment period. If you're attending school at least-half time, you may be allowed several years to repay.

- Subsidized Federal Stafford Loan. These are funds loaned to undergraduate and graduate students with a variable interest rate. There is also a grace and deferment period which means you may have extra time to pay the loan before you're charged penalties.

- Federal Direct Student Loan and Family Education Loan (FFEL). These low-interest loans are available for students and parents. Under the direct loan program, the federal government makes the loans. Under the FFEL, private organizations such as banks, credit unions and savings and loan associations make the loans.

  To confuse you even more, these loans are either subsidized or unsubsidized. Subsidized loans are awarded on the basis of financial need. Unsubsidized ones are not. You can receive both subsidized and unsubsidized loans as long as they're from the same program, either the Direct Loan or the FFEL.

For more information on financial aid—the what, why, when, where and how—write or call:

Federal Student Aid Information Center
P.O. Box 84
Washington, D.C.   20044
1-800-4-FED-AID (1-800-433-3243)

State Aid Programs

State aid programs differ from state to state and work much like federal aid programs. For more information, ask your guidance counselor or call your State Department of Education.

School Financial Aid Office

Many colleges, universities and vocational schools have a financial aid office which offers their own student aid programs. You'll probably need to turn in an application and financial statement every year.

Contact your college, university or vocational school financial aid advisor for further information on what's available and how and when to apply.

Other Special Funds

Your high school guidance counselor can help you find aid in other places, too, like civic organizations (Kiwanis, Rotary, Zonta, The Lions Club), 4-H, Girl and Boy Scouts of America and associations related to your field of study, like the American Medical Association or the American Bar Association.

Also, don't overlook the armed services. The Reserve Officers Training Corps (ROTC) is another source of federal monies. In the ROTC, you can earn while you learn. Go down to the local U.S. Armed Forces Recruiting Office for more information. Sometimes, too, Army, Navy, Air Force and Marine personnel visit juniors and seniors at the high school.

Many programs are also available for adults who want to continue their education, veterans, reserve and national guard members, single parents, those of certain ethnic origins (such as Indians), and students wishing to pursue degrees in specific areas.

You might as well camp in your guidance counselor's office in your senior year, because just as you figured, if you want more information on financial aid programs, that's where you'll need to be.

I don't know where to start!

Some states, through the Department of Education, have a computerized database that provides both state and national aid resources. (Use of this system may carry a small fee.)

Okay, I've decided to go to college. Where do I begin?

Your counselor can let you know the appropriate dates, fees, tests and deadlines to apply for scholarship and financial aid applications. However, you can use the following checklist as a guide:

Junior year:

- start thinking about colleges and write away for information
- take courses that will help you prepare for college
- take the PSAT
- find out if you have any chances at earning a scholarship

Senior year:

- take the ACT, SAT or Achievement tests if you haven't already done so. Request applications from the colleges your interested in and start working on your personal essay
- line up people to write letters of recommendation (teachers, coaches, counselors, employers)
- send in your applications to colleges
- get a FAFSA (Free Application for Federal Student Aid)
- get all your financial records together, fill them out and mail them to the school of your choice
- complete all forms on time and neatly—so people can read them
- keep a complete copy of records, instructions, deadline dates, forms submitted and letters
- call to make sure the colleges received all your application materials

Some Last Minute Advice . . .

Being able to finish high school speaks for more than your abilities in English or math. Your diploma says a lot about you as a person. It says you have what it takes to be a success in life. It says you have the guts and self-discipline to stick with something no matter how hard or how boring you think it gets sometimes.

If you're at risk of dropping out or have already done so, check out alternative education programs which can help you gain the skills needed to get back in school or get a job that matches your talents and desires.

If you don't finish high school, at least work towards getting your GED (General Education Development). The GED is as good as a high school diploma. No matter how old you are or how you did in school, there's always the GED.

The test covers five areas: writing, reading, social studies, science and math. At least one in five people in this country finish high school through the GED, and almost 75% of them pass the test. It may help you get a better job or help you get into college if and when you decide that's for you. If you want to know more, call free: 1-800-62-MY-GED.

. . . And Some More

Continuing your education isn't all about knowing what you want to do. It's about learning skills that will help you become whatever you want to be. In fact, most people don't have any idea what they want to do until after they experiment with different courses and activities.

If you decide to wait to go to college, it's never too late to start. The average age of a community college student is 29.

One thing that might help you decide how much and what type of education you need is finding out what the fastest growing job markets are and planning accordingly.

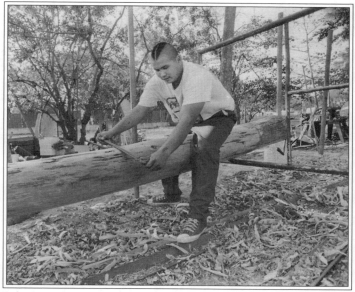

Kirk Condyles, Impact Visuals

What else is there besides college?

Take your pick. There are many programs available that combine school with real-world work. Depending upon the program, you could earn money, on-the-job training and work experience, a high school diploma, certificates of mastery of job skills, and an associates degree at a community college.

Vocational-technical programs, or "voc-tech," help students gain the skills they need for the job force or for college with hands-on and in-depth classes.

Here are a few examples of voc-tech courses:

- animal science
- automotive service
- cosmetology
- electronics
- drafting

- health services
- computers and information processing

School-to-career or school-to-work programs combine time in the classroom with real time on the job. They are made possible through partnerships between local businesses and your school, and include technical training programs, apprenticeships, internships, externships and other cooperative programs.

There are also career-tech opportunities for people who are challenged because of a handicap, lack of money, poor grades, imprisonment or weak English language skills.

Youth Employment Training Programs

If you're between the ages of 16 and 21, see if your area has youth employment training programs. These programs usually offer a little bit of everything: training in job search techniques (interviews, job application and resumes), summer and year-round job placement, as well as challenge camps, computerized reading and math labs, alternative education opportunities and vocational training.

Enlisting in the Army, Navy, Air Force, Marines or Coast Guard has given many young men and women a full-time job with the chance to earn money, receive technical or medical training and, in some cases, launch a lifelong career (and retire after only twenty years of service). Committing a few good years to the service may also help you earn credits or financial assistance toward a college degree.

Each of these armed services divisions also has part-time opportunities in the reserves. In the reserves, you can hold down a full-time job or attend college, while gaining the benefits of technical training and being paid for part-time duty.

The National Guard is like the reserves with the same part-time opportunities available in your home state.

Call the following free numbers for information and the location of the recruiter nearest you, or go down to your local recruiting office for the real detail.

U.S. Armed Forces: 1-800-USA-ARMY
U.S. Air Force: 1-800-USA-AIR F
U.S. Navy: 1-800-USA-NAVY
U.S. Marines: 1-800-MARINES
The Coast Guard: 1-800-424-8883

You might also check with the National Job Corps at 1-800-733-5627 who will refer you to the training center nearest you. The Job Corps offers GED and job training in such areas as health care, data entry, sales, construction, food services, accounting, clerical and science.

Volunteering is also a great way to prepare for future employment. You get on-the-job training, a chance to sample a possible career and solid references. Many volunteers even find jobs with the agencies they served for free.

All of these options will help you gain marketable skills and solve the old problem of: "I can't get a job without experience, and I can't get experience without a job."

For more information on any of these opportunities, guess who to call? That's right, your high school guidance counselor. You're catching on fast.

What kinds of careers are going to be hot in the '90s?

Jobs for the future will be in the areas of: health care, international finance, research science, the environment, telecommunications, social work, computers and the information superhighway (the Internet).

Please explain the Internet...so I can understand it.

The Internet is a network of computers that connects hundreds of millions of people together and allows us to move information around the world. That's where the Internet gets its nickname: the information superhighway.

To get on the Internet, you need a computer, a modem (the computer's idea of a telephone), and a phone line. Then, for a fee, you can subscribe to services which will put you "online."

Let's say you want to zip a message to a friend. Whether they're across the room or across the world, you can do it in seconds on the Internet's electronic mail or "e-mail." You can also "chat" or talk back and forth with that person. You can even join online discussion groups which are called "bulletin boards" or "forums."

The Internet can hook you up to thousands of other computers for doing research, shopping, reading newspapers and magazines, studying or testing your skills at video games.

Beware! Not everything on the Internet is so cool. Since the Internet has no owner, no one checks out the information before you see it, and there is no honor code. Thieves can steal private information off your computer. Stalkers and child abusers search the the Internet looking for their next victim. Discussion groups and pictures sometimes involve intense sex and violence. Some games have "viruses" which can destroy information on your computer. (There are people working on solutions to these problems, with the goal of making the Internet safe for all users.)

How do I go about looking for a job?

Whether you're looking for a job for the summer or for a career, here are some good ideas.

- Network. Let everyone know you want a job: friends, family, neighbors, past employers, teachers, counselors and others. Ask them what kind of jobs they think match your skills and interests. This is known as "networking".

- Talk to people who do the kind of work you want to do. Call employers in the industry that interests you. Ask to schedule a meeting to talk about their company and/or tour their facilities. Watch some of the employees at work and ask them about job duties, working conditions, training requirements and job entry. (Employers sometimes hire employee referrals before they advertise job openings.)

- Hit the streets. Check the classifieds, school bulletin boards and the local Chamber of Commerce. Keep an eye out for help-wanted signs. If something sparks you're interest, drop off a cover letter and resume and fill out an application.

- Applications, resumes and cover letters are written communications that tell an employer about you. Be certain they are complete, truthful and easy-to-read. They should sell you to the employer and tell why you are the best person for the job.

A resume (pronounced "re-zoo-may") is usually one typewritten page which briefly describes your education, work history and other skills.

The school or public library career resource centers have materials on "how to" write resumes and cover letters and answer difficult questions in interviews.

- Employers often ask for references. Try to provide at least three (but no relatives, please). References should be written by people who know your abilities such as teachers, former employers and other adults. Be sure to get permission to use their name, address and phone number in your job search.

- Collect samples of your work that fit the type of job you're looking for—artwork, charts and graphs from reports or papers you did for class, certificates of honor or special skills, and writing samples.

- Be realistic about the salary, days and hours, and position you expect. Many "first" jobs are in the fast foods or other retail sales industries which usually pay minimum wage or slightly above. Also, you may have to work nights and weekends.

- Make sure you have a social security number. If you don't have one, check the yellow pages for the Social Security office nearest you and get one.

- If you don't get the first job you apply for, don't give up. Go over the interview session, so you can do better next time. Keep trying until you get a job that's right for you.

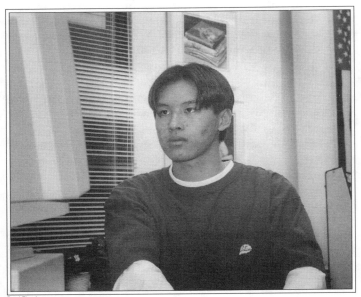

Brad Fleming

What are employers looking for when they hire people?

In the next 10 years and beyond, employers are going to be looking for people with 10 special qualities. Can you find yourself in this list?

1. Problem solvers—people who look for every option to solve a problem and don't go around complaining or blaming others.

2. Sifters and sorters—people who use their brains to make sense of the puzzles in the workplace, who know how to research and apply what they learn.

3. Heads that focus on the bottom line—workers who are out for results.

4. People who speak and write well, who can get their point across clearly using the best choice of words and correct grammar and spelling.

5. Team players who can listen, work well with others and want to help everyone win.

6. People who welcome new technologies and figure out ways to use them to reach the company's goals.

7. Idea people who are creative and try new ways of getting the job done.

8. Leaders who have insight into what the future may bring and who have self-confidence and pride in themselves and their own judgment.

9. "Surfers on the third wave"—learners who understand how fast change occurs and can handle it well.

10. Organizers and developers—people who can motivate and manage others and are good at directing and producing the best products and services.

(ADAPTED FROM: THE PRYOR REPORT)

How can I prepare for an interview?

You only have one chance to make a first impression. The interview can make or break you with an employer.

- Find out as much about the company as you can. The employer will be impressed that you took the time to find out. (Don't ask your mother, brother or a friend to call the company to find out either. That's a sure sign you can't do even the easiest job on your own.)

- Blow your own horn, without being cocky. Focus on your school work, special skills you might have and past work successes.

- Listen and build your answers on what the interviewer says.

- Talk about what you can bring to the job and the company.

- Bring your resume or a fact sheet listing your education, experience, social security number and references.

- Go alone! Dress for success.

- Be friendly and polite to everyone you meet—keep eye contact and give a firm handshake.

- Practice reading and comprehension, math, typing and other skills beforehand. Some employers give tests to help pinpoint qualified applicants, including personality tests. Try to relax in order to do your best at test time.

- After the interview, go home and put a second resume together—one that details how your skills are perfect for the specific job you're applying for.

- Keep a record of the companies and the dates you applied for work, and follow-up each one with a call or visit.

When I work either a part-time or full-time job, will I have to pay taxes?

Depending upon how much money you earn, you may be responsible for state and/or federal income taxes. The amount you must earn to be subject to taxation may also change from year to year.

Employers will ask you to sign a W-4 form for taxation purposes when you go to work for them. If you have questions about how to complete the form, ask your parents and your employer for help.

Is there anything else I should know?

Depending upon your age and the state you live in, there might be certain laws affecting your job.

These guidelines involve work hours, breaks and the types of jobs that kids your age can have. In some states, for example, you might not be able to work in jobs that call for hazardous or dangerous work (like washing the outside windows on a tall building). There may also be limits on your working where alcohol is sold or made.

These laws are made to protect you from injury or illness at work. You can find out from your employer what laws might affect you on the job.

Any tips for continued employment?

- always be on time
- show up for work every day
- dress neatly
- make an effort to get along with other employees
- be willing to do lots of different jobs
- stay on the given task
- arrange dependable transportation

Above All, Have Fun

My hopes for the future would be that one day a Willy Wonka Factory would be open to the world for visiting, and that Disney World would expand even further. The reason I say this is because people sometimes forget about having fun or relaxing. Enjoy life, you only live it once.

TRISHA, 17

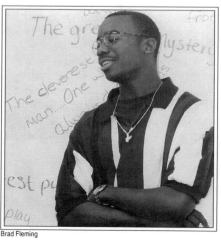

Brad Fleming

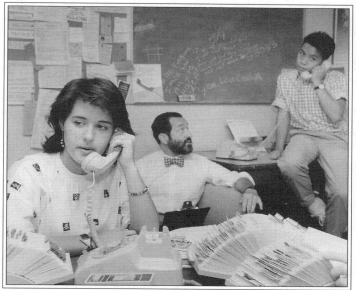
AP/Wide World Photos

12

People You Can Count On

Need help? Don't be shy. Getting help as soon as you can may keep a small problem from becoming big. Start by talking with your parents. You might be surprised what they know in their old age. Clergy, relatives and friends are good listeners, too, as well as your school's guidance counselor.

As you're searching for answers to your questions,

don't forget the yellow pages of the phone book. All agencies have phones, and the call probably won't cost you a dime. "Let your fingers do the walking" under the following headings:

Adoption Services	Employment
AIDS	Government
Alcoholism	Health Services
Associations	Human Services
Birth Control	Hospitals
Churches	Medical Services
Clinics	Mental Health
Clubs	Physicians
Counseling Services	Psychologists
Counselors	Religious Orgs.
Crisis Intervention	Schools
Dentists	Social Services
Drug Abuse	Youth
Education	

If you're not sure which agency to call, give it your best guess. Even if you're wrong, the person you speak with can probably point you in the right direction.

Shop around until you find a person or place you trust. Ask what services they provide and if there is any cost. Many agencies offer free services. If not, and you don't have any money, they may still be able to help. You may qualify for free services or a reduced free. Ask which services are directly available to you and which require the approval of a parent or guardian.

Different agencies can offer you counseling, shelter, health care testing and treatment, food, clothing, prenatal care, education, information, protection, adoption, financial and legal support and more.

Self-help groups, like Alcoholics Anonymous (AA), Narcotics Anonymous (NA), Alanon and Alateen hold meetings in a variety of places and at different times. To find out where a meeting is being held, or for more information on attending a meeting, try checking your local newspaper.

Free Helplines

There are several national helplines manned by trained counselors who can offer you information, one-on-one counseling and referral to community and state services.

If you don't get what you want or need on the other end of the line, don't give up. Call another number and another until you find someone who can help you. (The list that follows is just a small sample of what's available.)

You can talk freely with the counselors on these "crisis lines" because they have taken an oath to keep all calls private. However, in some states, if a counselor thinks you might do yourself or someone else harm or that abuse has occurred, they'll try to get your permission to call an ambulance or police officer.

Remember, the people you talk with can give you information, but they can't make up your mind for you. In the end, you'll have to make the decision that's best for you.

Medical Emergencies

Most towns and cities have 911. It's not an 800 number, but it's free, and the people who answer are trained to help in all kinds of medical emergencies.

Any Problem, Big Or Small

Third Level Crisis Intervention

Whatever is bothering you, call the local Third Level Crisis Intervention (you can usually find their number in the phone book under "Crisis Intervention.") They not only provide 24-hour counseling and suicide intervention, but can tell you where to go in your town or neighborhood for more help.

Boys Town National Hotline: 1-800-448-3000

If you have a concern or a problem you can call the Boys Town National Hotline, anytime of the day or night, for information, counseling and the names of places you can go in your own community for support. (Even though it's called the "Boys Town" Hotline, girls and parents can call it, too.)

Childhelp—IOS Forresters National Child Abuse Helpline: 1-800-4- A CHILD

No matter how old you are, no matter what time of day or night it is, if you're unhappy at home, at school or in relationships, there's someone to talk with at Childhelp. Maybe you or a friend need help to stop abuse at the hands of a babysitter or parents. You can even ask questions about sex, pregnancy or running away. Counselors can give you real-life suggestions for coping with a bad situation, and even hook you up with local professionals and services. Childhelp is also good for parents with concerns or anyone who needs to report abuse.

Youth Crisis Hotline: 1-800-HIT-HOME

Depression, sexuality, pregnancy, gangs, suicide, abuse...you name it, the Christian counselors on the Youth Crisis Line can offer counseling and referral to a local shelter or church 24-hours-a-day.

The "9" Line: 1-800-999-9999

The 24-hour "9" line offers counseling, information, and referral to local resources to both kids and parents in need. Counselors are ready to help in the case of someone who is suicidal, a runaway who needs shelter or those who abuse drugs and alcohol.

Children's Rights of America: 1-800-442-HOPE

"Need help? There's hope." Suicide, self-esteem, gangs—whatever the problem, the counselors on this national youth crisis hotline can help 24-hours-a-day. Children who are victims of abuse or anyone who believes a child is being abused should call the HOPE line.

For Runaways

The National Runaway Switchboard: 1-800-621-4000

If you or someone you know is on the run or thinking about running, this hotline is open all day, every day, for counseling or information about nearby services and shelters. They may also be able to help you arrange a free way back home. (Mom and dad can receive counseling at this number, too.)

Children of the Night: 1-800-551-1300

Lonely, frightened, homeless? You don't have to be. Call the counselors on this free, 24-hour helpline for comfort or referral to nearby shelters and health care services.

For Pregnancy, STDs and AIDS

National AIDS Hotline: 1-800-342-AIDS

Call the AIDS hotline, 24-hours-a-day, for information on how to prevent HIV/AIDS and referrals to clinics and hospitals where you can be tested, counseled and treated for HIV/AIDS. They'll also help you find financial, legal and medical support services.

The National STD Hotline: 1-800-227-8922

If you want information or need to be tested for any STD, the people on the end of this hotline can direct you to clinics or hospitals in your area (Monday-Friday only).

HIV/AIDS Treatment Information: 1-800-448-0440

Call this free number for information, counseling and referral to local HIV/AIDS services (Monday-Friday only).

National Life Center Hotline: 1-800-848-5683

Pregnant and scared? Call the Life Center Hotline anytime of the day or night for a referral to local agencies that provide counseling, testing, shelter, prenatal care, AIDS testing and maternity and baby clothes.

For Drugs And Alcohol Abuse

Alcohol and Drug Helpline: 1-800-821-4357

For help with a drug or alcohol problem, call the Helpline. Counselors answer calls around the clock and can "just talk" or direct you to a nearby place for counseling or treatment.

Cocaine Helpline: 1-800-COCAINE

For answers and referral about cocaine addiction, prevention and treatment, simply call this free helpline 24-hours-a-day.

For Child, Partner Or Elder Abuse

National Council on Child Abuse and Family Violence: 1-800-222-2000

This helpline provides information, assistance and counseling referrrals with regard to child, spouse/partner and elder abuse.

National Organization for Victim Assistance: 1-800-TRY-NOVA

If you are a victim of abuse, sexual assault or family violence, NOVA counselors are on-line around the clock to offer crisis counseling, information and referral to local programs and services.

EMERGENCY NUMBERS

Police/Sheriff _____

Fire Department _____

Family Doctor _____

Hospital _____

Crisis Intervention _____

Poison Control _____

U.S. Coast Guard _____

Search & Rescue _____

Other _____

_____

MEDICAL AUTHORIZATION

Parents: when you are away from home or travelling out-of-town, leaving proper medical authorization with your local hospital in the event of an emergency can be a life-saver for your child. Your consent legally authorizes physicians and surgeons to provide all of the necessary medical, surgical and hospital care your child may need.

The consent form should include information on your child's birth date, medical history, allergies, immunizations, family physician and insurance. Have the document notarized, keep a copy at home and give one to your local emergency department to keep on file. In your absence, make sure your child receives immediate and quality medical care . . . and give yourself a little peace of mind.

Bibliography

Get It? Got It. Good! is a product of years of investigation into some of the best articles, books and minds in the field of adolescence. This bibliographic selection is just a sample of what is available to help the next generation . . . as well as those of us who strive to understand and inspire them.

Creighton, Allan, and Paul Kivel. *Helping Teens Stop Violence.* Alameda, California: Hunter House, 1992.

Eyre, Linda and Richard. *Teaching Your Children Values.* New York, New York: Simon & Schuster, 1993.

Leman, Dr. Kevin. *Smart Kids, Stupid Choices.* Ventura, California: Regal Books, 1987.

Peterson's Summer Opportunities for Kids and Teenagers. Princeton, New Jersey: Peterson's, 1996.

Rubin, Nancy. *Ask Me If I Care.* Berkeley, California: Ten Speed Press, 1994.

Slap, Dr. G.B. *Teenage Health Care.* New York, New York: Pocketbooks, 1994.

White, Barbara, and Edward Madara, eds. *The Self-Help Sourcebook.* Denville, New Jersey: American Self-Help Clearinghouse, St. Clares-Riverside Medical Center, 1994.

Zerbe, Dr. Katheryn. *The Body Betrayed.* Washington, D.C.: American Psychiatric Press Inc., 1993.

Index

CAROL NOËL

Carol Noël has been a featured writer, lecturer and television newscaster in the health care field for more than 15 years. In addition to the national edition of *Get It? Got It. Good!*, Noël personally works with community coalitions throughout the United States and Canada to customize the teenage guide for their area. Noël resides in Northern Michigan with her husband, Brad, and their three children.

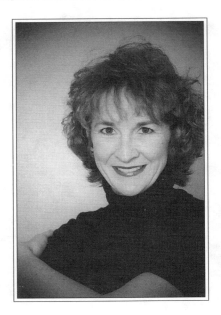

HOW TO ORDER

To order additional copies of the national edition of *Get It? Got It. Good!* or for information about customizing the teenage guide to reflect the needs, values, and resources in your community, call or fax your request to:

1-800-551-0124

or write to:

Carol Noël
Serious Business, Inc.
2909 DePew Road
Petoskey, MI 49770

A discount schedule is available for quantity purchases.

Signed copies are provided upon request.